THE

Rosemary Conley lives in l... business partner, Mike Rimm...... mary Conley Enterprises.

A qualified exercise teacher, Rosemary has worked in the field of slimming and exercise for twenty years, but it was in 1986 that she discovered by accident that low-fat eating led to a leaner body. Forced on to a very low-fat diet as a result of a gallstone problem, not only did Rosemary avoid major surgery but her previously disproportionately large hips and thighs reduced dramatically in size. After extensive research and trials her *Hip and Thigh Diet* was published in 1988 by Arrow Books. This book and its sequel, *Rosemary Conley's Complete Hip and Thigh Diet*, have dominated the bestseller list for four years and have sold in excess of 2 million copies. *Rosemary Conley's Hip and Thigh Diet* has been translated into five languages, including Hebrew and Greek. Subsequent titles, *Hip and Thigh Diet Cookbook, 1 & 2, Inch Loss Plan, Metabolism Booster Diet* and *Whole Body Programme*, have all been instant number 1 bestsellers.

Rosemary has travelled the world promoting her books, and her *Hip and Thigh Diet* has been number 1 in New Zealand, Australia, Canada and South Africa. She has appeared on numerous radio and television programmes world-wide, including the Ray Martin Show in Australia and the Wogan show in the UK. Since 1990 Rosemary has had her own series on network BBC 1 television.

In 1991 her *Whole Body Programme* video was launched by BBC Video. It too became a number 1 bestseller, topping the UK video charts for many months. It is to date the bestselling fitness video ever to have been released in this country. Further of her videos include *Whole Body Programme 2, Whole Body Programme 3 – Aerobics and Beyond, 7-day Workout* and the *Top To Toe Collection*.

Rosemary is now accepted as the leading authority in the UK on weight and inch loss. When asked why she has achieved so much success she says, 'It's simply because my diets and exercise work for ordinary, real people.'

Rosemary is a committed Christian and has a daughter, Dawn, by her first marriage.

Rosemary Conley's

COMPLETE HIP AND THIGH DIET

ARROW

This edition published by Arrow in 1993

9 10

Copyright © Rosemary Conley 1989

The right of Rosemary Conley to be identified as the author
of this work has been asserted by her in accordance
with the Copyright, Designs and Patents Act, 1988

First published in Great Britain by Arrow 1989

Arrow Books Limited
Random House UK Ltd, 20 Vauxhall Bridge Road, London SW1V 2SA

Random House Australia (Pty) Limited
20 Alfred Street, Milsons Point, Sydney,
New South Wales 2061, Australia

Random House New Zealand Limited
18 Poland Road, Glenfield
Auckland 10, New Zealand

Random House South Africa (Pty) Limited
PO Box 337, Bergvlei, South Africa

Random House UK Limited Reg. No. 954009

A CIP catalogue record for this book
is available from the British Library

Papers used by Random House UK Limited
are natural, recyclable products made from wood grown in
sustainable forests. The manufacturing processes conform to
the environmental regulations of the country of origin.

ISBN 0 09 911011 3

Phototypeset by Intype, London
Printed and bound in Great Britain by
Cox & Wyman Ltd, Reading, Berkshire

Contents

Acknowledgements

I would like to acknowledge with grateful thanks the readers and followers of both my original *Hip and Thigh Diet* and the subsequent *Complete Hip and Thigh Diet* who so kindly wrote marvellous letters telling me of their success on the diet, and those too who so thoughtfully completed questionnaires, which gave me a great deal of valuable information. Special thanks must go to those dieters who, having lost very significant amounts of weight, sent their 'before' and 'after' photographs for use within my TV programmes and who allowed me to quote from their stories here. I am also very grateful to those who submitted recipes for inclusion in this book. Without all these wonderful people this book would not have been written.

A warm thank-you as well to the following: JVF Consultants Ltd, whose expertise enabled us to reproduce on our computer the data from the questionnaires; my editor, Jan Bowmer, particularly, for her continued help, encouragement and support throughout the lifetime of the *Hip and Thigh Diet*; Dennis Barker, for producing such eye-catching covers; and Judy Collins for her help in sub-editing this latest book. Special thanks must also go to my secretary, Diane Stevens, not only for her endless hours of typing but also for her thoughtfulness and total co-operation.

Introduction

Dear Reader,

In January 1988 my *Hip and Thigh Diet* was first published and it was followed, a year later, by the *Complete Hip and Thigh Diet*.

The latter book included an extended diet and a great many testimonials confirming the effectiveness of this revolutionary diet plan, which I had hit upon completely by accident in February 1986 when diagnosed as having a gallstone problem. I was forced on to a low-fat diet, which not only enabled me to avoid major surgery at that time but also had the extraordinary side-effect of reducing my hips and thighs by a great many inches. I developed the diet which provided the basis for my *Hip and Thigh Diet* books.

At that time I had no idea that the book would remain in the *Sunday Times* bestseller list for five years. Along with other titles that I subsequently published, my books regularly enjoyed the number 1 position. At one point I had four titles in the top ten at positions 1, 2, 3 and 7! In November 1991 the *Sunday Times* decided to drop diet books from their general paperback bestseller list, perhaps because they were fed up with my books appearing on it with such monotonous regularity. I was, however, informed that *Complete Hip and Thigh Diet* was still riding high in the *real* list! In mid 1992, diet books were reinstated under the 'manuals' section, and at the time of writing, *Complete Hip and Thigh Diet* is at number 3.

I think it is reasonable to assume that the reason a diet book continues to sell consistently in such high numbers and for so long a time is simply because *it works*. I continue to receive thousands of letters from satisfied dieters who are astounded at the results they have enjoyed. The letters and completed questionnaires arrive from all corners of the world – the *Hip and Thigh Diet* has been a number 1 bestseller in five countries.

I followed the publication of *Complete Hip and Thigh Diet* with the *Inch Loss Plan*, the *Metabolism Booster Diet* and the *Whole Body Programme*, all of which have been number 1 bestsellers. However, there does seem to be a certain unique quality about the *Hip and Thigh Diet* which appeals to the general public and has consequently enabled its formula to reign as the *supreme diet* (despite the fact that the later books are, I feel, particularly strong in their message and effect). With the benefit of continuing correspondence from its followers I have been able to extend my research into the effectiveness of the Complete Hip and Thigh Diet and I felt it was appropriate to update the book and include the latest, more extensive statistics, coupled with some inspirational testimonials which offer very special words of encouragement for anyone thinking of embarking on a diet. I have also extended the menus as, during the last five years of following the diet continuously myself, I have learned and developed many new ideas and techniques for producing tasty meals. I have also been fortunate enough to be given additional recommendations by fellow-dieters. The menus that I have included extend far wider than previously and incorporate budget, as well as gourmet, suggestions. The 'vegetarian section' has been considerably expanded in order to cater for the increasing numbers of non-meat-eaters. This book also incorporates a section on exercise which was not included in the previous edition of my *Complete Hip and Thigh Diet* book, thus now providing a truly complete hip and thigh programme.

Diets are forever being criticized as being ineffective in the long term. Just prior to revising the *Complete Hip and Thigh Diet*, I had the privilege of being invited as a guest on the Wogan Show. My appearance coincided with the publication of a report in America that stated 95% of dieters regained their weight and many ended up weighing more than they had before embarking on their diet. Understandably, the effectiveness of my diets was questioned, and I welcomed the opportunity to deny vigorously that such statistics would be applicable to *my* dieters.

When I decided to expand and update *Complete Hip and Thigh Diet*, I determined to establish the diet's long-term results. My only way of establishing these facts was to write to those dieters whose weight details appeared in my earlier book and who had completed the original questionnaire. These same dieters had received a second questionnaire back in 1989 and a third at the end of 1991.

The response was very heartening. A staggering 40% of dieters had actually *maintained their weight loss over the five-year period*. A further 24%

11

had increased their weight *loss* during that period and maintained it thereafter, 8% of whom had actually doubled their weight loss. A further 12% had gained only a fraction – less than 25% – of their original weight loss. (Remember, the American survey reported 95% regained it all.) A further 8% had regained between 25% and 33% of their original weight loss and 12% had regained 33% or more of their original weight loss. Only 4% actually weighed more after the five years than they had when they started the diet. There was no doubt that the evidence proved conclusively that followers of my diet within this trial group had dramatically changed their eating habits with the effect that 76% of dieters had been able to maintain their weight, or their weight gain had been so insignificant as not to affect their size or general health. Against the reported 95% failure rate of most other diets, there is little doubt that the Hip and Thigh Diet is in a class of its own. I am not aware of any other diet author who has instigated such an investigation and published such long-term results.

The reason for this astounding success is simply that anyone who seriously followed the diet did actually enjoy the effect of a re-education of their palate which enabled them to change their eating habits. Not only that, if they did so for themselves the chances are that they did it for their families, too, thus enhancing their relatives' chances of enjoying better health and a longer life. There was, for example, an instance within my trial group where the husband had dieted alongside the wife and he had managed to lose 5 st (31.8 kg) of unwanted weight. You can well imagine the improvement to their general well-being as a result of the two of them drastically reducing in size.

The Complete Hip and Thigh Diet works in the long term because it actively re-trains your eating habits. Dieters soon get used to preparing their food in a different way and they find that after a short time following the low-fat regime they no longer miss the fat. Certainly the increased sense of well-being far outweighs any feeling of initial deprivation. When the dieter looks in the mirror and sees his or her shape returning to that he or she once enjoyed years ago, and experiences an energy level to match, there really is no argument. Often the husband follows the example of the wife when he sees what delicious food she is eating and then the children follow suit as the whole family realizes that this is the way to better health and more energy. It doesn't take long before low-fat eating becomes a way of life.

We are constantly being reminded by the various health programmes and authorities that a low-fat diet is the way forward for a healthier future. From the thousands of letters that I have received, and particularly from those who have enjoyed enormous benefits to their health as a result of following the low-fat diet, it is clearer than ever that this is the route we should be taking. Ironically, it took vanity – a desire to *look* better through reducing the fat around our hips and thighs, or around our tummy or our backs (wherever the fat is deposited) – to spur us into action. For years we had been told to eat less fat in the hope that it would help prevent a potential heart condition, but the 'it won't happen to me' syndrome prevailed and few people took heed of this advice. However, dieters soon became excited when they could see emerging the cosmetic benefits to their shape.

When I myself embarked on a very low-fat diet rather than undergo major surgery, I discovered the fantastic side-effect which can only be described as a miracle. My disproportionate pear-shaped body began to change shape and inches fell off my hips and thighs for the first time in my life! The members of my exercise classes pleaded with me to share the diet with them and, amazingly, after only a few weeks they enjoyed the same results – shedding those inches previously impossible to shift.

It was at this stage that I tested the diet further with a team of volunteers recruited through local radio stations and 120 men and women followed the diet for an eight-week trial period. It then became obvious that it wasn't just large-hipped figures that benefited. Those with a top-heavy, 'busty' figure lost weight from their busts, and those with a more roly-poly figure lost it from around their tums. I believe this diet is so effective in shedding inches from our body's waste grounds because the body utilizes the highly nutritious food, rather than storing it as reserves of fat as is the case with most high-fat junk food. In the Department of Health and Social Security's Report 28 on 'Diet and Cardiovascular Disease', it suggests that *everyone*, regardless of weight, sex, age or condition, could benefit from reducing their fat intake by about one third. I read in one book that we need only six grams of fat a day, and yet most people in the Western world consume a daily average of 130 grams. My diet does not stipulate that slimmers eat anywhere near as few as six grams, just considerably less than the average daily intake. On the Maintenance Programme, the fat allowance is increased, although it still remains lower than the amount we have been used to.

Nutritionally we need fat for energy and certain vitamins. Since these fat-soluble vitamins can be stored in the body, there is little risk of deficiency for the duration of the diet. I nevertheless recommend that everyone following this or any other diet take a multivitamin tablet each day to make sure that they are eating sufficient vitamins.

Just three weeks after the first *Hip and Thigh Diet* book was on sale, letters began flooding through my letterbox. Words like 'incredible', 'fantastic', 'staggering', and 'amazing' were used to describe the effect of the diet on readers' bodies. 'I've regained my youthful figure after twenty years'; 'I just wouldn't have believed it could have happened, let alone so quickly and so easily!' It was truly wonderful to hear how well the diet was working for everyone.

Also, among the many letters I received, there were many requests for more vegetarian menus and packed lunches. Readers also outlined the benefits to their health that this diet brought them. Arthritics enjoyed greater mobility and less pain; heart patients enjoyed real improvements in their condition; many found that digestion improved and symptoms of PMT disappeared. Also, not surprisingly, gallstone sufferers enjoyed significant relief. The results of 250 questionnaires showed that 89% of respondents felt healthier on this diet.

In response to countless requests, I produced an exercise audio cassette and, more recently, a new exercise video for hips and thighs, which contains the most effective exercises to help tone up this difficult area. This *Hip and Thigh Diet* video, part of my *Top To Toe Collection* published by the BBC, I recommend people to buy in preference to the original. Also, there is a Postal Slimming Course for those who feel they need personal support. See the last page of this book if you wish to consider applying for any of these aids. We just want to help you to achieve the kind of figure you've always dreamed of. Exercising has never been more fun; and dieting has never been simpler: there's plenty to eat and no calories or units to count – just incredible results to enjoy.

With very best wishes.

Rosemary Conley

PS It is always advisable to check with your doctor before embarking on this or any other diet programme. Most people will benefit from undertaking exercise, but do check with your doctor if you feel that there may be some doubt as to your suitability.

Measurement Record Chart

Date	Weight	Bust	Waist	Hips	Widest Part	Top of Thighs L	R	Above Knees L	R	Upper Arms L	R	Comments

Measurement Record Chart

Date	Weight	Bust	Waist	Hips	Widest Part	Top of Thighs L	Top of Thighs R	Above Knees L	Above Knees R	Upper Arms L	Upper Arms R	Comments

Measurement Record Chart

Date	Weight	Bust	Waist	Hips	Widest Part	Top of Thighs L	R	Above Knees L	R	Upper Arms L	R	Comments

Measurement Record Chart

Date	Weight	Bust	Waist	Hips	Widest Part	Top of Thighs L	R	Above Knees L	R	Upper Arms L	R	Comments

1
'It works! It really, really works!'

'Thanks a million. It works! It really, really works!' read the letter from Lorna Cowley, just one of many I received shortly after the publication of my *Hip and Thigh Diet* in January 1988. Cynthia Wall wrote: 'I never thought I'd be writing to anyone saying "your diet is wonderful" but it is, and I am!'

Claire Davison reported: 'I have lost a stone (6.4 kg)! And have never in all my fat life (I was 11 st 1 lb [70 kg] at ten years old) eaten so much food, or felt so well or had so much energy. I feel like a teenager again (I'm fifty-six years old).' Stella H. wrote: 'I started your Hip and Thigh Diet last August and between August and November lost 4½ st (28.5 kg). A low-fat diet and more exercise has meant that I am continuing to lose weight and I am absolutely thrilled . . . I cannot remember when I last felt so well and don't bother weighing any more. Compliments are more than sufficient to tell me the diet (change of lifestyle) is continuing to make a difference . . .'

Audrey Bewley from North Yorkshire wrote: 'I have been following your Hip and Thigh Diet and every word is true – the weight has gone from the most stubborn parts of my body. I truly love the diet.' During the eight-week trial period that Audrey

21

followed the diet she lost 1 st 2 lbs (7.3 kg). She and her husband have continued with the diet and, not only has Audrey maintained that original weight loss, she has actually decreased her weight by a further 1 st 7 lbs (9.5 kg), resulting in a grand total of 2 st 9 lbs (16.8 kg). She has maintained this new weight of 9 st 1 lb (57.6 kg) for over a year now. She wrote: 'You will be pleased to hear that my husband who has always been heavily built has almost reached his goal ... he has lost nearly 5 st (31 kg) ... I don't know his measurements, just that he looks so good!'

I *knew* my diet worked. It has worked for me and it has left me in no doubt as to its effectiveness when my original trial team put it to the test. The results really were staggering. When the *Sunday Express* bought the serial rights to my book I was terribly excited. I never once doubted my diet's effectiveness but I knew it was not easy to convince the media. *This* diet was different. *This* one worked. *This* one was easy to follow. *This* one made you feel good – not irritable like most diets. And, yes, it really *did* reduce inches around those parts other diets didn't reach.

'Why hasn't anyone discovered the diet before?' I was asked many times during my promotional tour for the book. Funnily enough this type of diet *had* in fact worked before for others but they hadn't realized what was happening to their bodies. I was in an ideal situation, with all the circumstances just presenting themselves perfectly. Let me explain. When, in 1986, I was struck down with a gall bladder problem and faced imminent surgery, I was just winding up a business and about to become self-employed. I couldn't possibly take six weeks off to have my gall bladder removed, so I opted to follow a virtually fat-free diet. I was very determined and I did it! In my job as a slimming and exercise teacher I needed to wear skin-tight leotards and tights. At 5 ft 2 ins (1.57 m) I was not really overweight at 8 st 7 lbs (54 kg) but my enormous posterior and thunder thighs did make me look much weightier than I really was. Consequently, when these embarrassing areas began to slim down, but the rest of me stayed the same, my exercise students became inquisitive – eager that I should pass on my secret for their benefit! This I did and, yes, it worked for them too.

As I had already had several books published on the subjects of slimming, exercise and positive attitude, it seemed obvious that I should publish a book describing my new miracle eating plan. I realized that to convince the world at large (and my publisher) that my new diet worked, I would have to have detailed information on its success rate. As a regular broadcaster on local radio I asked listeners to try out the diet. They did and it worked for them as well. In fact 89% said they lost weight from the areas they particularly wanted to slim. It was so exciting to hear their comments, to see their diminishing measurements, to read how well they felt and how they never felt hungry. I just couldn't believe how positive everyone felt. It was wonderful.

My publisher was as excited as I was. Contracts were hastily drawn up and agreed, and four months later I had finished the book. I can remember posting it by registered post and thinking to myself – I *know* this is going to be a bestseller.

Two weeks after publication my book entered the non-fiction paperback bestseller chart – at number 1. I just couldn't believe it! It stayed there for the next week – dropped to 2, then 3, then up to 1 again where it stayed for over six months. The publishers kept reprinting and the readers succeeded in losing their weight and inches and telling their friends.

After about a month I began receiving letters – lots and lots of very encouraging letters. The readers were saying they just couldn't believe that the diet was in fact working just as I had said it would. They couldn't believe the change in their shape. They couldn't believe that this diet worked even though they seemed to be eating much more food than normal. It was their total shock at its effectiveness that prompted them to write. Here are some extracts from their letters.

Pam Irwin wrote:

'Initially when I read your book I thought "this is too good to be true", but I've followed your diet plan for eleven weeks now (not too rigidly – having breaks for birthdays and weekends away!) and have lost 22 lbs (10 kg). I have also lost 4 ins (10 cm) from my bust, 4 ins (10 cm) from my waist and an amazing 6 ins (15 cm) from my hips and 3 ins (7.6 cm) each from my thighs, and I haven't found it a problem or that I'm giving up anything. Never have I lost so much so easily and quickly! I also feel 100% better in myself and my skin and hair have never been in such good condition!'

Jane F. from Kenilworth wrote:

'I imagine you have hundreds of letters every day telling you how fantastic your diet is and lots of different stories. I never thought I would be sitting here writing a letter about a diet, but it is incredible!

As a young teenager I was quite slim, but at seventeen years old I got married, then pregnant and weighed in at over 15 st (95 kg). I started going to the clinic with my son and joined their slimming club and exercise afternoon. It took a long time and after I finished at the clinic I continued to diet on my own and was very pleased that on my twenty-first birthday I weighed 10 st 12 lbs (69 kg).

When I was twenty-six years old my husband left me and I very easily slipped into the habit of eating and eating. I then met up with a lad I had gone out with as a schoolchild and have been with him ever since. I have been "on" and "off" diets for years, but have put on more weight than I have lost. My boyfriend was quite happy and, as he puts it, "likes me with a bit of fat". My mother died last year and instead of not being able to eat like some people I worked my grief away by eating constantly. In November, I weighed 13 st 9 lbs (86.6 kg). It was then that I read your book and my sister and I started your diet on 5 November. By 24 March I was down to 11 st 2 lbs (71 kg), feeling great, and down three sizes in clothes. I had reached what seemed an ideal weight and went on to your Maintenance Programme. At the beginning of the diet this was the part I was dreading – either putting my weight back on, or the thought of always having to watch what I eat. But surprise, suprise, it's easy!

It's now 18 April and, guess what, I weigh 10 st 12 lbs (69 kg) – the same weight as when I was twenty-one years old, and I look and feel twenty-one years old again. All I really wanted to say is thank you so very much for a fantastic diet which is so easy.'

I sent a questionnaire to Jane and her inch losses were dramatic. She had lost 6 ins (15 cm) from her bust, waist and hips, 5½ ins (14 cm) from the widest part and 3 ins (8 cm) from each thigh. She added:

'I have been on the Maintenance Programme for several weeks now. I don't think I could eat as I used to ever again. It seems almost impossible to put weight on. In fact I'm eating a little bit extra to make sure I don't lose any more for the time being.

Thank you so very much for your wonderful diet. Absolutely fantastic! I now weight 10 st 6 lbs (66 kg).'

Jill Erikson wrote:

'I am writing to you because you have done so much for me and my family. Today I attended Outpatients for my six-monthly check-up. The nurse was staggered by my 24 lb (11 kg) weight loss. My performance on the blowmeter, or whatever they call it, surprised the consultant, particularly as I was not taking my two drugs – a heart pill and a steroid for breathing. I have started to play golf again for the first time in 12 years. My golf handicap is coming down! Until Hip and Thigh I was literally dying, wanting to retire, everything was an effort and I couldn't wait to go to bed.

I am fifty-six years old, a bronchial asthmatic

(lifelong, with several pneumonia bouts), I have had ankylosing spondylitis for forty years and in 1966 I had a major road traffic accident and was hospitalized for a year.

Some seven years ago I decided I had had enough of the medical profession. I tried all types of diets and read up on nutrition, vitamins, minerals, etc. There were marginal improvements, but gradual physical deterioration; no energy, no enthusiasm and I was very depressed about galloping old age. *Hold everything*! My eighteen-year-old daughter, wanting to lose a few pounds, brought home your *Hip and Thigh Diet* book and the rest is history.'

One of the criticisms I received as a result of the publication of my *Complete Hip and Thigh Diet* was that I didn't include any details about significant weight losses. This was because my research was based on only eight weeks' dieting on the part of most of my volunteers. Obviously, as the years have passed, I have been able to learn of many more who have lost very considerable amounts of weight. Ann Brown is a perfect example. She wrote:

'I have never had so much success so quickly as on this diet. The results are so immediately noticeable. The last stone (6.35 kg) was quite hard to lose, but I just was very strict with myself. It really was easy and as my husband did it with me (he needed to lose a stone), it made it fun planning meals too. Two years is not really long to transform myself totally for the rest of my life. I continue to follow the diet and I would like ultimately to weigh under 9 st (57.2 kg).'

At the time of returning her completed questionnaire, Ann had lost 7 st (44.5 kg) – a far cry from the 16 st 7 lbs (105 kg) she weighed two years earlier. With her 5 ft 4 ins (1.62 m) height and large frame, 9 st 7 lbs (60.3 kg) enabled her to look very slim in the photograph that she sent me. Her inch losses were dramatic. Ann lost 10 ins (25 cm) from her bust, 8 ins (20 cm) from her waist, 10 ins (25 cm) each from her hips and widest part, 6 ins (15 cm) from each thigh and 4 ins (10 cm) from each knee. Her figure now measures an enviable 36–26–36 ins (91–66–91 cm).

During the early part of 1992 my second television series was screened on BBC 1. One of the joys of such a programme was the opportunity to meet many people who had enjoyed the benefits of my low-fat diets and had reduced their weight dramatically. We regularly showed 'before' and 'after' pictures, which were of great inspiration and encouragement to countless viewers. The success of three of these was particularly outstanding and I felt this new edition of *Complete Hip and Thigh Diet* wouldn't be complete without their stories. The three had followed the Complete Hip and Thigh Diet to achieve their stunning weight losses.

Susan Randall wrote:

'It's great! This diet really does work! After being tubby as a child and always a bit overweight as a teenager, I went to being extremely overweight after having my two children. At the age of twenty-six, 5 ft 10½ ins (1.86 m) tall and weighing in at 16 st 1 lb (102 kg), I was depressed and I felt and looked awful. An old friend (who was also tubby at school) recommended your Hip and Thigh Diet after she had lost several stones on it and so, with her success as my motivation, I gave it a try.

A year later and 5 st 5 lbs (34 kg) lighter, I am delighted. I feel great, my confidence has increased and I actually wore a size 12 straight skirt this week – something I have never done before. My measurements have gone from 44–38–50 ins (112–96–127 cm) to 36–28–38 ins (91–72–97 cm), along with 6½ ins (16 cm) from thighs, 6 ins (15 cm) from above the knees and 3 ins (7 cm) from the arms – quite a change. I still have about 7 lbs (3 kg) to lose, but I'm confident that it will go and that I can keep it off. My husband joined me on the diet to give me encouragement and lost 1½ st (9.5 kg) into the bargain.

I felt I had to write as I hope my success will help somebody else to shed those unwanted stones.'

I wrote to Susan and asked her to complete a questionnaire. The results are: Over a period of fifty-six weeks, Sue had lost 5 st 7 lbs (35 kg). At 5 ft 10½ ins (1.86 m) tall, she looked very slim at 10 st 5 lbs (65.7 kg) when she came on my programme. Sue had lost 8¼ ins (21 cm) from her bust, 10 ins (25.4 cm) from her waist, 12 ins (30.4 cm) from her hips, 6 ins (15.2 cm) from each thigh and 4 ins (10 cm) from each knee. She now had an enviable 36–28–38 ins (91–72–97 cm) figure that was very trim for her large-size frame, which is indicated by the fact that she takes size 8 shoes.

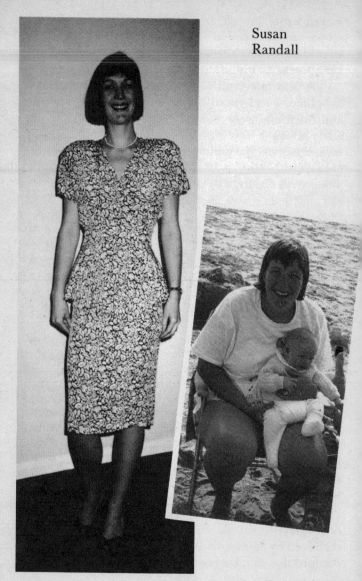

Susan
Randall

Susan wrote:

'This diet has become a way of life to the family – my children eat the same meals as we do and so it is fairly easy for us to maintain our weights. I feel really healthy and so much more confident than I have for a long time. I hope by writing to you someone else will be inspired by my loss and achieve what I have done.'

I first met Kathryn Orr when she came along with her husband to watch one of my television programmes being made in the Metro Centre at Newcastle in early 1992. She introduced herself and bowled us over with the news that in the last eighteen months she had lost 8 st (50.8 kg)! Initially Kathryn stuck strictly to the Hip and Thigh Diet losing 42 lbs (19 kg) in twelve weeks but then she modified it to her own liking, just eating very low-fat food and regularly exercising to one of my workout videos. In the following fifteen months she lost another 5 st (32 kg), finally reaching her goal of 10 st 5 lbs (65.7 kg). When we met I couldn't believe Kathryn had ever been overweight let alone once weighed over 18 st (114 kg)! So impressed were we by her story that we invited Kathryn along to another programme recording a few weeks later so that she could inspire our viewers.

I asked Kathryn to complete a Hip and Thigh Diet questionnaire. She had lost 12 ins (30 cm) from her bust, 12 ins (30 cm) from her waist, 12½ ins (32 cm) from her hips and 14 ins (35.5 cm) from her widest part. Prior to following the diet Kathryn admitted to frequent bingeing. This had now ceased completely. Despite the fact that previously she had

31

tried more diets than she cared to remember, on this one she felt healthier, her cellulite had reduced, the condition of her hair and nails had improved and she had actually enjoyed following the diet. One of the main reasons for this was the fact that she could eat so much more than on most other diets.

At the end of the questionnaire Kathryn wrote:

'The Hip and Thigh Diet worked for me because I liked the freedom of choice and I never felt bored or hungry, which is very important when you have a lot to lose. I found I was losing weight from the areas I wanted to lose from most and this encouraged me to keep going . . . I now feel like a new person. My life has changed so much for the better and I feel fitter than I have for years.'

We were alerted to another outstanding success story when a set of photographs and an accompanying letter particularly caught our eye.

Mr A.L. and his wife had been married for five years and having gone through the normal fertility tests they were told that they could not produce children of their own. Whilst this news came as a great disappointment they came to terms with the facts and decided that adoption was the next best option.

The local adoption panel considered their application but then the couple were dealt another cruel blow. Their application was refused because Mr L. was overweight – 6 st (38 kg) overweight, in fact. Needless to say, they were devastated.

The reason for the overweight factor resulting in the refusal of their application is the health risks involved from being overweight. Any child who is

Kathryn
Orr

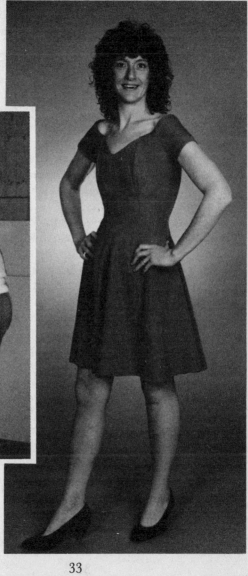

available for adoption has already had a difficult start in life and, understandably, every effort is made to ensure that its second chance of a secure and stable future is as good as possible.

Mr L. was given six months to shape up before the panel made their final decision. As it happened, Mr & Mrs L. already had a copy of my *Hip and Thigh Diet*. The same day they were told of the ultimatum, Mr L. started the diet – in earnest. Mrs L. was distraught when she realized her husband had to lose 6 st (38 kg) in that time. His previous attempts to lose weight had yielded little or no results. But never before had they had such an incentive to reach a goal.

After twenty-four weeks Mr L. had lost a stunning 6 st 7 lbs (41 kg)! He now weighed 13 st 9 lbs (87 kg), which was ideal for his 6 ft 3 ins (1.9 m) height. His figure had reduced from 46–40–43 ins (117–102–109 cm) to a very trim 40–32–40 ins (102–81–102 cm). Mr L. was not alone in his success: his wife lost 2 st (13 kg) at the same time! She is now a petite 7 st 8 lbs (48 kg).

So impressed were the adoption panel by the obvious determination shown by this couple, and the fact that Mr L.'s weight now offers no threat to his health, they have decided to accept Mr & Mrs L.'s application. It will probably take about a year before this deserving couple are handed their baby. I can't help feeling that words cannot sufficiently describe that anticipated moment of joy.

More dramatic weight losses are recorded on pages 60–65.

2
Binge no more!

In my previous books I deliberately avoided stating quantities of foods except those which contained fat, e.g. chicken, fish, meat. Fruit and vegetables are offered freely in the hope that slimmers will fill themselves and satisfy their hunger at the same time as breaking that *negative* habit of counting calories or units. I believe calorie counting leads to binge eating. We are able to cope with a restricted diet for most of the day, but four o'clock arrives, we've munched our way through most of our daily allowance and the prospect of a slim-line evening is just too much. We nibble a little to start with, then it turns into a wholesale binge. We throw in the towel and say, 'Oh well, I'll start properly tomorrow!'

I used to binge terribly – I have now stopped completely. Since I have followed my very low-fat diet I find I can eat such a volume of food, I don't feel deprived as I used to when dieting previously. So the fact that I don't specify how big that jacket potato should be is quite deliberate. If having a 12 oz (350 g) potato (which is quite big) means you won't have a binge later, eat it and enjoy it. After a while you will find that as you are allowed one every day if you wish, you don't really *need* such a big one. Gradually you will find yourself selecting food portions much more sensibly. You will feel more relaxed about eating. Your confidence in your will power will gradually increase and you will feel much better about yourself. The same rule applies to your portion of rice or pasta. Eat enough to satisfy yourself.

There is nothing more negative for someone who is trying to reduce their weight than getting up from the table feeling not quite full. If you do this, you will feel deprived and are most at risk to temptation. I usually cook extra vegetables so that I can fill myself up with them if I'm still feeling peckish.

I have an enormous appetite which constantly shocks those who eat with me. I eat as much as most men and when you realize I am quite small at 5 ft 2 ins (1.57 m) I am living proof that this diet *does* work. One word of warning here – if your progress on my diet is really too slow, it is likely to be your portion size that is to blame, so bear this in mind.

Comments made by readers in their lovely letters to me suggested that they had been able to change their previous bad eating habits completely since following my diet. I wanted to know exactly why this was so, and my comprehensive questionnaire was offered to anyone interested in giving me more details of their progress. In the last four and a half years, I have received over a thousand completed questionnaires. The data from these has been computerized and the results are included in this book.

I asked if they had ever binged before following my diet and 78% said they had, whilst the remainder had never done so. I then asked if they had binged at all whilst following the diet and 24% said they binged occasionally whilst 74% said they didn't binge at all, 1% said they had continued to binge and the remainder didn't answer the question.

The whole concept of bingeing is quite extraordinary and something that interests me greatly. Bingeing is, I believe, the greatest cause of overweight. Yet most bingeing is done whilst trying to diet! This sounds like a contradiction, but so often someone goes on a diet to lose a few pounds and before they know it they've actually *gained* weight. Just after I was first married I had only 14 lbs (6.4 kg) to lose. I lost 12 (5.4 kg) of them, had a binge, felt cross with myself and panicked – left the slimming group I attended feeling ashamed and in five weeks regained all that I'd lost plus another 14 lbs (6.4 kg)! How often has that happened to slimmers? Millions of times – all because they felt so deprived whilst following the diet. So why did the vast majority of those following my Hip and Thigh Diet *not* binge?

Of those who completed my questionnaire, 63.6% felt their success on this diet, compared with previous diet failures, was attributable to the fact that they could eat so much more on this diet.

I asked my volunteers what they considered were the most enjoyable aspects of my diet. I offered ten options plus space for additions and asked them to award marks from 1 to 10 in order of preference, marking their favourite aspect with 1 point, and their least favourite with 10.

This was the result, in order of preference:

1. Plenty to eat.
2. No calorie counting.
3. Freedom of choice of menus.
4. No weighing of food.

5. Having three meals a day.
6. Eating lots of fruit.
7. Eating as many vegetables as I liked.
8. Eating potatoes.
9. Eating bread.
10. Having a three-course dinner.

So it is clear to see that lack of hunger and the plain simplicity of the diet were the keys to its success.

Armed with this information, we can now think logically about when we normally binge. I believe we wage a personal war between ourselves and a diet. We feel hungry and a normal slimming diet says, 'Too bad, you've had your calories – tough!'

We say, 'I don't want to feel hungry. Why should I feel hungry? Blow it, I'm going to eat and I'm going to eat what I want!' And off we go for the highest calorie food we can get our teeth into. In fact, it becomes almost like a race to see how much food we can ram down before the diet 'claps us in irons' again. During a binge we really want to make the most of it – sultanas, raisins out of the baking cupboard, ice cream out of the freezer, cheese from the refrigerator, bread and jam, biscuits (even the ones we don't like) – *anything*! We never think, 'I'll have egg and chips', because that would take too long. We want food *now*. Also, we think we're only going to have just this little . . . but it's never a 'little' anything, because it's a nasty, deceptive, slippery slope which we tumble down, faster and faster, away from all reason or common sense. We are often not truly conscious of what we are doing. Afterwards we are furious with ourselves. If you've ever binged – you know what I mean.

So, avoiding binge eating is the key to success if we want to stick to a reducing diet; and want to achieve our goal and stay there!

One reader, Linda Wood, wrote to me, saying:

'I am a lot more confident about myself because I know my weight will continue to come off, as I am eating so much more healthily. In fact, I don't feel as though I'm "rushed" on this diet; I feel this diet is a whole new way of eating for me. It certainly works for me, I feel tons better for it, and have lost all my guilty feelings about bingeing.'

This diet does in fact prevent a lot of the feelings of hunger and deprivation which lead to bingeing. And if you can cure bingeing, you can be assured that you'll keep around your ideal weight for ever. As Miss J. W. wrote:

'My once regular evening binges seem to have been eradicated for ever as my mental attitude has changed for the better. So thank you for helping me to feel like a spring chicken!'

3

'Yes – this diet really *does* slim hips and thighs!'

After my own experience of the diet and seeing the results of my initial trial team there was no doubt in my mind that this diet *does* slim hips and thighs. During my various promotional tours that have included Australia, New Zealand, Canada and South Africa, I was constantly questioned by interviewers as to the *real* effect of the diet. 'But surely you lose weight from problem areas if you slim for long enough anyway,' they would say. Yes, that's true, but you would also lose weight from areas you didn't want to slim, such as your bust.

I was determined to show that my diet *did* work, and I was lucky enough to have plenty of people to back me up. Followers of the diet were so overwhelmed at their success that they wrote telling me of their experiences and miraculous inch losses; at every radio phone-in, someone rang in to say how brilliantly the diet had worked for them – losing inches exactly from where they wanted to.

Perhaps the best example of this was when I was in New Zealand. My publicist took me along to one of the local radio stations in Auckland where the presenter actually asked if the lady who had recently rung in with her weight loss story could possibly phone in whilst I was on-air. This was now my second visit to Auckland, and to this radio station, and since my previous visit the presenter had herself been on the diet. She had shed 2 st (12.7 kg) and the diet had become a regular topic for conversation on this live talk-back show.

Halfway through the forty-five-minute interview, Gay Smith telephoned. I couldn't believe my ears or my good fortune at being put in touch and, better still, being able to speak to her on-air. This remarkable lady had managed to lose 4 st 9 lbs (29.5 kg) since I had last visited. We chatted briefly on-air and I was given her telephone number so that I could contact her for a private chat later. But my good luck wasn't to stop here, as during our conversation I learnt that Gay was to fly to Sydney the next day to visit a nephew who was graduating from university. This coincided with my visit to Sydney, where I was to appear on the Ray Martin Show – a lunchtime version of the Wogan Show, and just as popular.

To cut a long story short, we were able to get Gay Smith on to that show with me, together with 'before' and 'after' photographs, and I had the delightful opportunity to meet Gay in person and to have a long and enjoyable chat. The two of us still correspond and during my last trip to Australia I hoped I would be able to meet up with Gay, but unfortunately there was no reply when I telephoned. I wrote her a card and this was her reply:

'Thank you for your card – sorry I missed you, but we were out of town for a few days. Yes, I have kept the weight off, I don't dare to do otherwise as too many people are watching me and after a lifetime of being overweight I still get a kick out of seeing myself in the mirror. It is still hard to believe. I hope you and your family are all well as this leaves us here.

Lots of love and best wishes always, Gay Smith.'

Here are some more extracts from just a few of the many, many letters I have received:

Nurse Janet Farrar wrote:

'Not only have I been impressed with this diet and its results; my colleagues (I am a nurse) have been so amazed that many of them have followed the diet, also with surprising results.

I have been teaching dance and exercise classes for some years, and in spite of all the exercise I do and have done, I have never been able to reduce my enormous thighs significantly – until now. I intend following the diet and maintenance programme and spreading the good word to as many people as possible!
PS   I am a whole dress size smaller now! Wonderful.'

Jo Hodgart wrote:

'Although I have not lost a great deal of weight I have lost inches, yet virtually none from my bust.'

On previous diets Jo said her bust completely disappeared.

Mrs J.P.N. wrote:

'As you will see from this questionnaire, I could hardly be described as "overweight" being 7 st 9 lbs (49 kg) to begin with. However, I did have pads of fat on my hips which looked like saddlebags which developed during my last pregnancy, over fourteen years ago. I had found this fat impossible to shift, even after practically starving myself at one stage – all I succeeded in losing at that time was my bust! So, when I heard about the Hip and Thigh Diet I decided to give it a go, although I was very sceptical that it would work. You can imagine how I felt when I could almost literally see this very unwanted fat disappearing in front of my eyes. I am delighted with the results. I must be honest and say that I didn't follow this diet to the letter, rather I adapted it to suit myself. There weren't too many three-course dinners for me – I found that simply too filling – but I did stick strictly to a low-fat diet, as I discovered which foods contained little or no fat, and I will keep to a low-fat diet in the future.'

Angi White wrote:

'As many other readers of your book have remarked, when trying other diets in the past all the weight has either disappeared from the face or the bust which is most discouraging as: 1. You are told that you look ill, and 2. I can't afford to lose weight from my bust.

With your diet all the excess weight is disappearing from the places I've always wanted it to – from my lower half. It feels great to be able to wear tight-fitting jeans and skirts again without feeling the pinch!'

Margaret Bowman wrote:

'This is a letter I've been meaning to write since I achieved my goal of losing 2 st (12.7 kg) in the winter. In February 1991 I decided to try your diet for a week. Now, seven months later, I am still "on the diet" – that is, not dieting but continuing with eating healthily and sensibly. I started off at 10 st 6 lbs (66 kg) and now weigh 8 st 7 lbs (54 kg) – down from size 14 to size 10 – and, yes, the fat from my "rear-end" has now gone and I am slimmer than I was when I got married at nineteen years old. I have found that eating out occasionally and eating forbidden foods occasionally doesn't automatically mean a weight gain, providing one's normal daily eating plan includes food low in fat.

Thank you once again for turning me from a frumpy middle-aged mum into a mini-skirted energetic person!'

Kathleen Proctor was one of my most enthusiastic correspondents. Having lost 1 st 6 lbs (9 kg) in nine weeks, her figure was transformed. Kathleen wrote me a detailed account of her weight loss campaign and backed it up with the most remarkable photographs. A keen cyclist, her 'before' photograph showed extremely ample thighs. Having shed her excesses, she sent me an 'after' photograph showing her thighs in the shape any model would be delighted to possess. Not an inch of flab, or cellulite – just beautifully contoured slim thighs.

Kathleen wrote: 'As it was my thighs I particularly wanted to reduce I measured only them accurately, but my other areas I had measured some weeks earlier, and I couldn't seem to shift inches from them.'

Kathleen also suffered from severe pain from several gallstones and was waiting to be admitted into hospital.

'I've followed your low-fat diet and I've achieved the following:
A) Reduced my pain by over 50%.
B) Lost all my excess weight.
C) Lost inches from the right places.
D) Kept the weight I didn't want to lose.
E) Feel healthier and fitter.
F) My skin looks better.'

She went on to say:

'I've regained my teenage figure, I'm now thirty-seven. I knew I'd lose weight, but never like I've done on this Hip and Thigh Diet . . . My thighs and bottom are so slim, I'm absolutely ecstatic. What a way to go on holiday! Couldn't be better.'

And looking at Kathleen's photographs, I'm not surprised she's delighted.

Ann Burton wrote to me explaining that all her life she had wanted to lose weight from her hips – 'dieting usually meant losing it from my bust and waist only'. After reading my book she decided to give the diet a whirl. In seven weeks she lost 12 lbs (5.4 kg) and reached her goal.

'I was astonished at the amount of food I was actually eating and only very rarely did I feel hungry between meals. . . . In fact, I don't regard myself as being on a *diet* – I am eating sensibly and healthily. I have lost 2½ ins (6 cm) from my hips and 2½ ins (6 cm) from the top of my thighs.

I can now get into clothes which have always been too tight but, on the other hand, some of my clothes are now too large.'

Joanne Goulding wrote:

'I just thought that I would write and tell you how successful your Hip and Thigh Diet has been for me and to express my thanks to you for developing it.

As I was not really overweight or fat to start with I was quite amazed that I lost weight and in the right places.'

Joanne lost 1 in (2.5 cm) from her bust and waist, 3 ins (7.5 cm) from her hips, 3½ ins (9 cm) from her widest part, 2½ ins (6 cm) from each thigh and 2½ ins (6 cm) from around the top of each knee. At 5 ft 1½ ins (1.56 m) she was delighted to reduce from 8 st 7 lbs (53 kg) to 7 st 12 lbs (50 kg) – ideal for her height.

Valerie Cousins wrote:

'Your Hip and Thigh Diet has completely changed my life. I am only a small person (5 ft 2 ins [1.57 m] in fact) and was not terribly overweight at 9 st 7 lbs (60 kg). I now weigh 8 st 9½ lbs (55 kg). I have been on your diet seven weeks, but am determined to stay on it further. I am told I look years younger and it's all thanks to you. I am so grateful to you . . . I seem to have so much confidence since regaining my teenage figure.'

I asked Valerie to complete my questionnaire. By then her weight had reduced to 8 st 7 lbs (53 kg). It was good to see that Valerie had lost nothing from her 32 in (81 cm) bust, but her waist had reduced by 2 ins (5 cm) to 26 ins (66 cm). Her inch loss from her largest areas – hips and tops of legs – was a wonderful 4½ ins (11 cm) and 4 ins (10 cm) respectively, leaving her with youthful 35½ in (90 cm) hips. She commented:

'I am now able to put on my jeans; I feel like a teenager again. I have not stopped the diet as I wish to improve my figure further and you have given me the determination to do this. I have no intention of smothering my bread in inches of butter again – I have no wish to.
    This diet really has become a way of life for me.'

Barbara Jones wrote:

'This diet has produced such a noticeable effect, especially on the hips/thighs, that everyone has commented on it. Lots of people have gone out and bought the book as a result. I feel fitter and healthier and, I have been told, look younger. I have lost weight in proportion and although I am still somewhat overweight (I want to lose another 7 lbs [3.2 kg]), I have gained a balanced figure, which makes me look slimmer. I have previously

47

lost the same amount of weight, which I regained, but have never achieved my present shape. I have never felt the urge to binge or break my diet, although we have still socialized and gone out for meals, so I feel this time it will be easier to maintain my weight.'

Sharon Rice wrote:

'Before starting the diet I was slightly overweight, yet despite working out three times a week at the gym I was unable to shift any weight from my hips or buttocks; especially bad was the pad of fat that had accumulated around the hips and at the back of the hips. The gym instructor said it was the hardest place to shift fat from, but suggested some exercise which I had to do hundreds of "repeats" of. I persevered with the exercises until your book came along, and hey presto! With a combination of the diet and the exercises, the flab started to disappear.

The thing I liked most about the diet was the variety and amounts of food that I could eat. This fitted in perfectly with my weight-training, unlike other diets. I work out strenuously for 1½ hours, three times a week, so on the days that I wasn't training I'd eat "light" selections, i.e. lots of fruit and salad, then on training days when I needed something more filling, I'd opt for the "heavier" selections, i.e. bread, jacket potatoes, baked beans, etc. Following this routine I found the weight came off steadily, and has stayed off.

The other good thing is that although I'm no longer following the diet, I've found my eating habits have changed for the better. I don't miss butter in sandwiches – it's no longer necessary – nor my once-weekly portion of fish and chips – far too fatty. The hardest part is avoiding the "hidden" fats in biscuits, cream crackers, etc., but I am trying to re-educate myself.

My hair and skin have improved no end.'

Lynn Cook wrote:

'I now weigh 10 st 2 lbs (64.5 kg) and miraculously the weight has gone from all the right places. I have lost 2½ ins (6 cm) from my hips and 1½ ins (3.8 cm) from each thigh and 1 inch (2.5 cm) from my waist. When I have tried to diet in the past by counting calories, the weight was lost from the wrong areas and I didn't find the amount of food allowed satisfying enough. On your diet I am rarely hungry and find that I really enjoy the food.'

The following week Lynn completed a questionnaire, by which time she had lost another 2 lbs (1 kg) – making her loss 12 lbs (5.4 kg) in seven weeks. Her hips had slimmed still further from 41 ins (104 cm) to 38 ins (97 cm), her widest part from 42 ins (107 cm) to 39 ins (99 cm). She had lost only 1 inch (2.5 cm) off her bust, reducing it to 34 inches (86 cm). She summed up by saying:

'I think this diet has revolutionized my eating habits and I will be able to follow the maintenance diet permanently (with the occasional lapse such as when eating out, which I don't need to feel guilty about).'

How important that last comment is: don't feel guilty when you do dine out.

Janet Lea wrote:

'I would like to say a very big thank-you for giving me the inspiration to do something about my shape. I have always had a very definite pear shape throughout my life, and a big bottom which has always made me most unhappy; and I have always tried to exercise/diet in order to lose this shape. Although I have never been exactly overweight, I always found difficulty in buying clothes and remained a pear shape with a lot of cellulite around my thighs which was most unsightly in either shorts or bathing costumes. As I got older (I am forty-two) I found it increasingly difficult to diet and very often when trying to reduce my calorie intake, found I felt quite nauseous and not able to continue a diet for more than a couple of days. In fact over the past three or four years I had found it impossible to follow any diet at all, and had resigned myself to accepting I would always be pear-shaped.

I read an article on Rosemary Conley and was inspired by what appeared to be a kindred spirit. I thought I would give this diet my once-and-for-all best shot. To my surprise I found it easy to follow, most enjoyable, and was not hungry at all. Friends and colleagues at work were amazed at the loss of weight from my waist and hips as my shape had been a source of much comment – and indeed I still have difficulty in accepting that I am a slim size 12 as opposed to a lumpy 14. Friends are constantly remarking on my new shape.

Because I have a job as a secretary which naturally means sitting down a lot, I am amazed at how the cellulite has gone. My thighs are quite smooth in comparison to before and I would not now hesitate to wear shorts or a swimming costume and without constantly pulling down the legs to hide my lumpy thighs. I feel and look more attractive and I am very happy with my new shape.'

Janet lost 17 lbs (7.7 kg) in eight weeks, and lost 2 ins (5 cm) from her bust, 4 ins (10 cm) from her waist and hips, and 2½ ins (6 cm) from each thigh.

Veronica Jarvis wrote:

'I have felt so well and already can see how the inches are disappearing. Before I felt bloated and had no energy but now, even after a hard day, I no longer feel worn out. My thighs have always been like tree trunks and have never responded to any other diet I've tried. Although I would dearly love to lose more from that area, they do look a better shape.'

As I was reading through the original manuscript of this book before delivering it to my publishers in 1988, I received a questionnaire from Mary Hamilton and I just had to include her comments and statistical information because they were so good.

Mary lost 34 lbs (15.4 kg) in 14 weeks, she is 5 ft 2 ins (1.57 m) tall and now weighs 9 st 10 lbs (61.7 kg). She lost 2½ ins (6 cm) from her bust, 4 ins (10 cm) from waist, her hips and widest part, 2½ ins (6 cm) from her left thigh and 3½ ins (9 cm) from her right one. This is what Mary wrote on the back of her questionnaire:

'Ever since I had my tonsils out at the age of five, I have been fat. My lightest weight ever was 9½ st (60.4 kg). My heaviest was 11½ st (73 kg). That was when I tried your diet. My thighs were really enormous – in fact my husband used to say that if he could breed pigs with legs like mine he would make a fortune! Today is 26 June and I am down to 9½ st (60.4 kg) which is where I started from. Altogether, I have lost 2 st (12.7 kg) on this diet even though I have occasionally cheated. My thighs are still a bit heavy although I can now wear trousers without looking totally ridiculous. My aim is to reach 8½ st (54 kg) or possibly 8 st (51 kg) by which time my thighs should be normal – I hope.

The best thing is when people say to me, "You've lost some weight, haven't you." I feel very proud of what I've done. All the jokes about not stepping off high pavements because I'll bang my bottom are a thing of the past, thanks to your diet. Let's hope I can carry on and lose another stone (6.4 kg). Who knows, even I might get into a pair of size 10 slimfit jeans.'

When Veronica returned her third questionnaire to me, in 1992, she explained that she had maintained her weight without any difficulty up until November 1991, when she had to have an operation on both feet, which made her immobile for almost three months. Inevitably her weight crept up. Despite regaining 14 lbs (6.4 kg), she has now been able to reduce by another 7 lbs (3.2 kg) and is feeling much better already.

*

By asking readers to complete the questionnaire I was able to see clearly the evidence of inch loss from normally stubborn areas. And I received answers to many other useful questions.

An incredible 94% said they were surprised with their inch losses achieved on my diet. I asked the question, 'What was your reaction after following the Hip and Thigh Diet?' Over half (52%) were 'amazed', 27% were 'pleasantly surprised', whilst virtually all of the remainder (18%) felt 'satisfied'. Only 0.4% were disappointed.

The league table of parts of the body to reduce most significantly is as follows (some dieters ticked more than one area):

Hips and thighs	92%
Tummy	60%
Thighs	43.3%
Waist	43%
Bust	14%
Knees	7%
Arms and others	6%

By any stretch of the imagination this was a pretty staggering result. These figures are even better than those from my previous trials. As the diet detailed in the book was considerably extended from its original trial form it gave the slimmers more choice and accordingly a much greater degree of success.

It was interesting too that the 14% of volunteers who most wanted to lose inches from their bust did exactly that. You will see from the sample tables on pages 60–65 that we have included the final bust measurements. It is obvious from these details that only those with a large chest lost a lot of inches whilst those with a smaller figure lost, proportionately, significantly less.

It is also vital to realize that most of the inches lost from the bust measurement are not from the breasts themselves but from the back, where many women have a great deal of fat. There is no doubt that this diet gets rid of the fat on your body and if you haven't got fat on your breasts then you won't lose inches from the bosom itself.

The statistics from the returned questionnaires were computerized, enabling me to see average inch losses across the board. In arriving at the following set of figures no consideration was taken as to whether slimmers were male or female, fairly slim or very overweight, or whatever. A straight average calculated the following inch losses:

	inches lost	(cm lost)
Bust/chest	1¾	(4.4)
Waist	3	(7.6)
Hips	3⅙	(8.1)
Widest part	3¼	(8.2)
Thighs (each)	2⅙	(5.5)
Knees (each)	1⅓	(3.4)

The average weight loss was 2 lbs (1 kg) a week and the average length of time that these slimmers had followed the diet was ten weeks.

I think this is an amazing result, particularly because some of those following the diet admitted to being only fairly strict, whilst others only wanted to lose a few inches and very little weight. Any doctor would say that the ideal rate of weight loss is 1–2 lbs (0.5–1.0 kg) a week. This had worked out perfectly! However, as you will see in a later chapter, the best results were enjoyed by those who followed the diet very strictly.

Several of my correspondents continued to write and kept me posted of their progress. One of the most recent letters was from Sharron Johnson, the youngest of my original Hip and Thigh Diet trial team:

As one of the 'guinea-pigs' of the Hip and Thigh Diet it's hard to believe that five years has passed since it was first launched . . . I am so happy that it has become such a huge success; mainly because it is the only diet I know of that works and when you have been on it you no longer crave the foods you once did, enabling you to maintain your weight.

If your diet had not come along when I was seventeen years old, who knows what weight I could have been today. Even now, if I add a few pounds I know that I can bring my weight down again by going on the diet for a few days.'

I felt that Mrs K.B.'s comment summed up exactly what many would be thinking this year:

'I shall continue the diet in the hope of displaying my thighs on the beach this summer without embarrassment for the first time!'

Mary Coppins-Brown wrote:

'It is a joy and pleasure to be able to wear straight dresses without any hip and thigh bulges, and to use the last hole instead of the first hole on belts! Thank you for allowing me to share in your successful diet.'

On 7 May 1991 I received a letter from Hilary Youngman, who wrote:

'I have been on your diet for two and a half weeks and couldn't wait any longer before writing to you. I have lost 10 lbs (4.5 kg) already, absolutely painlessly.

Over the years my weight has crept up, in spite of diets (which never worked), until this year I reached 14 st (89 kg) and was feeling dreadful. If you are literally an answer to prayer, thank you very much.

My librarian daughter brought the book home for me and after two days I went and bought one for myself. I told my neighbour, who also bought one, started the diet six days ago and has lost 3 lbs (1.4 kg).

My goal weight is 10 st (63.5), which is what I weighed when I was married twenty-five years ago. My husband is delighted at my progress and utterly amazed when he looks at the plate full of food at the evening meal. I am 5 ft 8 ins (1.7 m), so hope to look willowy again, eventually.'

Just two months later Hilary wrote to me again and this is what she said:

'I wrote in early May after I had been on your wonderful diet for about three weeks. Thank you for your most encouraging reply. I must now let you know how many people have joined me on the diet and their incredible success.

My neighbour has lost the 1 st (6.4 kg) she wished to lose and is now happily watching me "fade away".

My husband, who has for the last year had stomach problems stemming from the removal of his gall bladder ten years ago, has been eating fat-free for the last four weeks. He has lost 8 lbs (3.6 kg) and his mini spare tyre but, more importantly, feels better and is eating a great variety of food, whereas his diet before was very restricted and most things upset him.

My mother, who will be eighty years old next week, spent a month with us in June after an unexpected trip to hospital when we thought we would lose her. While here she ate low-fat and, although at 10½ st (66.7 kg) for her 5 ft 8 ins (1.9 m) she was not overweight, she loved the meals. Two weeks after her return home, her hips, stomach etc. are very trim and she is absolutely bouncing towards her eightieth birthday.

A friend from choir has lost a whopping 2 st (12.7 kg) in eight weeks. She is looking so well and feeling it too. She wants to lose another 1½ stone (9.5 kg), so is continuing with the diet.

I have lost 23 lbs (10.4 kg) and am also feeling wonderful. I'll settle for losing another 25 lbs (11.3 kg), which will take me to 10½ stone (66.7 kg).

So, there are some very happy and newly healthy people in Blenheim, New Zealand.'

Hilary continued on the diet and on 15 September 1991 she wrote:

'We had a wonderful holiday in California and

Hawaii. I was able to fit into my bathing suit and swim (for the first time in years!). I even bought a pair of shorts and now have a suntan for the first time in years!'

On the following pages I give details of the actual weight and inch losses enjoyed by just a sample of those who completed my questionnaire. I have indicated the age group in each case. Names have been stated where permission has been granted. The tables show the inch losses achieved and the resulting bust measurements, and clearly show that if you have a small bust you do not lose a great deal from it on this diet.

Not everyone lost a lot of weight and some lost more inches than weight. For instance Kathleen Frake only lost 3 lbs (1.4 kg) but she lost 1 in (2.5 cm) from her bust, 4½ ins (11 cm) from her waist, 4 ins (10 cm) from her hips and 1½ ins (4 cm) from each thigh! In fact I often advise people not to be too concerned with the scales – but do take the time and trouble to measure yourself. With this in mind you will notice that I have included Measurement Record Charts at the beginning of the book (pages 17–20).

WEIGHT AND
INCH LOSS
STATISTICS

Name	Age group	Weeks on diet	Weight lost lbs (kg)	Inches lost from:			Inches
				Bust (cm)	Waist (cm)	Hips (cm)	Wides (cm)
Ann Browne	25–34	104	98 lbs (44.5 kg)	10 (25 cm)	8 (20 cm)	10 (25 cm)	10 (25 cm
Audrey Bushby	35–44	16	35 lbs (15.9 kg)	2 (5 cm)	6 (15 cm)	3 (8 cm)	–
Margaret Dominey	55–64	12	36 lbs (16.3 kg)	5 (13 cm)	4 (10 cm)	4 (10 cm)	4½ (11 c
Jeanette Froude	35–44	20	40 lbs (18.1 kg)	6 (16 cm)	6 (16 cm)	6 (16 cm)	5½ (14 c
Phillippa George	35–44	12	28 lbs (12.7 kg)	1½ (4 cm)	3½ (9 cm)	3½ (9 cm)	5½ (14 cr
Wendy Grant	25–34	20	40 lbs (18.1 kg)	3 (8 cm)	4 (10 cm)	5 (13 cm)	5 (13 cr
Grace Hickmott	65–74	22	50½ lbs (22.9 kg)	5 (13 cm)	6 (15 cm)	7½ (19 cm)	8 (20 cr
Mrs S.P.	35–44	24	84 lbs (38.1 kg)	12 (30 cm)	12 (30 cm)	14 (36 cm)	–
Therese Rundle	55–64	8	30 lbs (13.6 kg)	1 (2.5 cm)	3 (8 cm)	5 (13 cm)	3 (8 cm

Thighs	Knees R. (cm)	L. (cm)	R. (cm)	Bust measurement at end of diet ins (cm)	Height ft/ins (m)	Weight now st/lbs (kg)
(16 cm)	6 (16 cm)	4 (10 cm)	4 (10 cm)	36 ins (91 cm)	5 ft 4 ins (1.63 m)	9 st 7 lbs (60.3 kg)
(8 cm)	3 (8 cm)	–	–	33 ins (84 cm)	5 ft 4 ins (1.63 m)	8 st 13 lbs (56.7 kg)
/4 (6 cm)	2¼ (6 cm)	3½ (9 cm)	3½ (9 cm)	36 ins (91 cm)	5 ft 6 ins (1.68 m)	10 st 10 lbs (68 kg)
(8 cm)	3½ (9 cm)	1½ (4 cm)	2 (5 cm)	38 ins (97 cm)	5 ft 7 ins (1.70 m)	10 st 11 lbs (68.5 kg)
¾ (7 cm)	3 (8 cm)	2 (5 cm)	2 (5 cm)	37 ins (94 cm)	5 ft 9 ins (1.75 m)	10 st 8 lbs (67.1 kg)
(8 cm)	3 (8 cm)	1½ (4 cm)	1½ (4 cm)	36 ins (91 cm)	5 ft 4½ ins (1.64 m)	9 st 7 lbs (60.3 kg)
¼ (10.5 cm)	5¼ (13.5 cm)	2½ (6 cm)	2½ (6 cm)	38 ins (97 cm)	5 ft 6 ins (1.68 m)	10 st 12½ lbs (69.2 kg)
	–	–	–	40 ins (102 cm)	5 ft 8 ins (1.72 m)	13 st 10 lbs (87.1 kg)
(13 cm)	3 (8 cm)	1 (2.5 cm)	1½ (4 cm)	37 ins (94 cm)	5 ft 7½ ins (1.71 m)	11 st 8 lbs (73.5 kg)

Name	Age group	Weeks on diet	Weight lost lbs (kg)	Inches lost from: Bust (cm)	Waist (cm)	Hips (cm)	Inch Wid (cm
Jacqueline Storey	25–34	22	56 lbs (25.4 kg)	6 (15 cm)	6 (15 cm)	8 (20 cm)	8 (20
Miss N.W.	25–34	40	42 lbs (19.1 kg)	2 (5 cm)	3½ (9 cm)	7 (18 cm)	7 (18
Diane Wilson	15–24	37	88 lbs (40 kg)	7 (18 cm)	10 (25 cm)	15 (38 cm)	–
Alison Fielder	25–34	20	44 lbs (20 kg)	5 (13 cm)	8 (20 cm)	7¾ (20 cm)	9½ (24
Mrs M. Hughes	45–54	20	21 lbs (9.5 kg)	6 (15 cm)	8½ (22 cm)	5 (13 cm)	10 (25
Mrs W.A.	55–64	16	28 lbs (12.7 kg)	1 (2.5 cm)	4 (10 cm)	4 (10 cm)	5 (13
Mrs J.H.	25–34	20	28 lbs (12.7 kg)	3½ (9 cm)	4½ (11 cm)	5½ (14 cm)	7 (18
Claire Jones	15–24	8	12 lbs (5.4 kg)	2½ (6 cm)	2½ (6 cm)	5½ (14 cm)	5½ (14
Bridget McDonald	45–54	26	30 lbs (13.6 kg)	1½ (4 cm)	1 (2.5 cm)	6½ (17 cm)	7½ (19

Thighs L. (cm)	Thighs R. (cm)	Knees L. (cm)	R. (cm)	Bust measurement at end of diet ins (cm)	Height ft/ins (m)	Weight now st/lbs (kg)
½ (16 cm)	6½ (16 cm)	5 (13 cm)	5 (13 cm)	34 ins (86 cm)	5 ft 3 ins (1.60 m)	9 st 7 lbs (60.3 kg)
(10 cm)	4 (10 cm)	2½ (6 cm)	2½ (6 cm)	34 ins (86 cm)	5 ft 6 ins (1.68 m)	9 st 4 lbs (59 kg)
–	–	–	–	39 ins (99 cm)	5 ft 0 ins (1.52 m)	10 st 13 lbs (69.4 kg)
(13 cm)	4 (10 cm)	3 (8 cm)	3 (8 cm)	38 ins (97 cm)	5 ft 8 ins (1.72 m)	10 st 6 lbs (66.2 kg)
3½ (9 cm)	3 (8 cm)	2 (5 cm)	2 (5 cm)	42 ins (107 cm)	5 ft 4¾ ins (1.64 m)	14 st 7 lbs (92.1 kg)
2½ (6 cm)	2½ (6 cm)	1 (2.5 cm)	1 (2.5 cm)	34 ins (86 cm)	5 ft 9 ins (1.75 m)	10 st 0 lbs (63.5 kg)
4 (10 cm)	3½ (9 cm)	–	–	35½ ins (90 cm)	5 ft 7 ins (1.70 m)	10 st 8 lbs (67.1 kg)
2 (5 cm)	2 (5 cm)	1 (2.5 cm)	1 (2.5 cm)	36 ins (91 cm)	5 ft 4½ ins (1.64 m)	9 st 7 lbs (60.3 kg)
4 (10 cm)	4½ (11 cm)	2 (5 cm)	2 (5 cm)	34½ ins (88 cm)	5 ft 2½ ins (1.59 m)	8 st 10 lbs (55.3 kg)

| Name | Age group | Weeks on diet | Weight lost lbs (kg) | Inches lost from: | | | Inche |
				Bust (cm)	Waist (cm)	Hips (cm)	Wide (cm)
Mrs S.A.W.	25–34	12	28 lbs (12.7 kg)	1½ (4 cm)	4 (10 cm)	4 (10 cm)	3 (8 cm
Cathryn Fleetwood	25–34	34	68 lbs (30.8 kg)	5½ (14 cm)	8½ (21 cm)	11½ (29 cm)	–
Jackie Hunt	25–34	71	189 lbs (85.7 kg)	16 (40 cm)	20 (51 cm)	24 (61 cm)	–
Kathleen Frake	45–54	8	3 lbs (1.4 kg)	1 (2.5 cm)	4½ (11 cm)	4 (10 cm)	2 (5 cm
Fiona Duckworth	25–34	16	38 lbs (17.2 kg)	3 (8 cm)	3 (8 cm)	4½ (11 cm)	4 (10 c
Mr A.L.	35–44	24	91 lbs (41.3 kg)	6 (15 cm)	8 (20 cm)	3–4 (8–10 cm)	8–9 (20–
Hilary Youngman	45–54	10	22 lbs (10 kg)	3 (8 cm)	4 (10 cm)	7 (18 cm)	7 (18 c
Helen Chapman	25–34	13	26 lbs (11.8 kg)	4 (10 cm)	7 (18 cm)	4½ (11 cm)	5 (13 c
Imelda Dwyer	25–34	104	70 lbs (31.8 kg)	5 (13 cm)	6 (15 cm)	7 (18 cm)	10 (25 c

highs	R. (cm)	*Knees* L. (cm)	R. (cm)	*Bust* measurement at end of diet ins (cm)	Height ft/ins (m)	*Weight* now st/lbs (kg)
● cm)	2 (5 cm)	1 (2.5 cm)	1 (2.5 cm)	36 ins (91 cm)	5 ft 7½ ins (1.71 m)	10 st 5 lbs (65.8 kg)
/2 ● 4 cm)	5 (13 cm)	4¾ (12 cm)	5¼ (13 cm)	37 ins (94 cm)	5 ft 4 ins (1.63 m)	11 st 0 lbs (69.8 kg)
3½ ●4 cm)	14 (36 cm)	10 (25 cm)	9 (23 cm)	36 ins (91 cm)	5 ft 8 ins (1.72 m)	10 st 3 lbs (64.9 kg)
●/2 ● cm)	1½ (4 cm)	1 (2.5 cm)	1 (2.5 cm)	35 ins (89 cm)	5 ft 4 ins (1.63 m)	9 st 0 lbs (57.1 kg)
¾ ●.5 cm)	1 (2.5 cm)	1½ (4 cm)	1½ (4 cm)	38 ins (97 cm)	5 ft 7 ins (1.70 m)	11 st 7 lbs (73 kg)
● cm)	3 (8 cm)	1–2 (2.5–5 cm)	1–2 (2.5–5 cm)	40 ins (102 cm)	6 ft 3 ins (2.6 m)	13 st 9 lbs (86.6 kg)
5 cm)	2 (5 cm)	1 (2.5 cm)	1 (2.5 cm)	39 ins (99 cm)	5 ft 10 ins (1.77 m)	12 st 3 lbs (77.6 kg)
¼ 3 cm)	¾ (2 cm)	¾ (2 cm)	1 (2.5 cm)	35 ins (89 cm)	5 ft 6 ins (1.68 m)	9 st 9 lbs (59 kg)
½ 11 cm)	5 (13 cm)	4 (10 cm)	4 (10 cm)	32 ins (81 cm)	5 ft 6½ ins (1.69 m)	10 st 7 lbs (66.7 kg)

4
The 'Tum and Bum Diet' for men

Some weeks after the original diet had been published I spoke to the Associate Editor of the *Sunday Express*. He said, 'I've been following the diet since you gave me a copy and I've lost 13 lbs (5.9 kg) and have lost inches exactly from where I wanted – just around my middle. In fact we men have renamed it the "Tum and Bum Diet".' Men do not have to worry about jodhpur thighs as that isn't normally where they put on excess weight – it is almost always around the middle. Whilst women have 'thunder thighs' or 'child-bearing hips' men suffer from a 'beer belly'.

On my previous trials only three men had participated, but this time I had lots of husband-and-wife teams who wrote to me quite spontaneously about their successes. In my replies (I replied to everybody who wrote to me) I asked if they would be kind enough to complete a questionnaire. The results were wonderful. Here are just a few.

Evelyn Eaglestone wrote telling me how she and her husband both felt the diet was ideal for them, 'We just cannot believe that we can tuck into such lovely food and still lose weight.' Evelyn's husband, Stanley, lost 15 lbs (6.8 kg) in eight weeks and lost 4 ins

(10 cm) from around his waist (he only took this measurement). Evelyn lost an amazing 21 lbs (9.5 kg), losing 1 inch (2.5 cm) from her bust, 2 ins (5 cm) from her waist, 3 ins (7.5 cm) from both her hips and widest part and 2 ins (5 cm) from her thighs. She said, 'Other diets have left me feeling so low and hungry that I've said "Life is too short to suffer this", and that "I would rather die of over-eating than starvation", but with your diet you've got the best of both worlds. Eat plenty *and* lose weight! What more could anyone wish for?' She continued:

'I must tell you what really made me realize I was so overweight. All winter I went round the house in a bright green track-suit (extra large). One day I opened the door to the milkman. "You look smart in your green," he said. "Yes," I said, "kidding myself I'm the green goddess!" "Well," said he, "I was thinking more of the Jolly Green Giant!" We both rolled up laughing but it made me think.'

Mrs J.B. explained that her husband suffered from high blood pressure and joined her on the diet. 'He lost 17½ lbs (8 kg) and felt better for it.' She also explained that she had lost weight a couple of times before with the help of a slimming club but whilst she might have lost more weight on these occasions it didn't seem to go from the areas she *wanted* to slim. Family and friends always commented on the fact that her face looked drawn, but not this time. 'In fact my sister asked me which diet I'd been following and went out immediately and bought your book.'

Margaret Craven wrote:

'Since Christmas 1990, I kept thinking I really ought to do something about my increasing figure. My skirts and trousers were getting tighter and clothes just did not look so good any more. So, after talking to my partner's sister Pat, who also wanted to lose weight, we enrolled in a "Swing into Shape" class, held weekly at a school near us, which lasts for 2 hours per week. After searching for a leotard which looked *fairly* reasonable and "Max Wall" tights, off Pat and I trotted. We found the routines fairly easy to follow, and after a hot bath on returning home, no aches the next day! But, oh the second day! Muscles ached where I didn't know muscles existed, but I felt so *different*, invigorated, so we have both looked forward to each weekly session, sometimes twice weekly.

Pat then bought your *Whole Body Programme* video and *Complete Hip and Thigh Diet* book, and in only a week she had lost 6 lbs (2.7 kg) and inches from where she wanted to. As it was my birthday, my partner Fred bought me the video and book also, and after reading it through, the fridge and freezer suffered a severe refurbishment as I ruthlessly discarded any food on the forbidden list and passed it on to my grateful parents.

Within a week, Fred and I had lost 7 lbs (3.2 kg) each. Fred lost 3 ins (8 cm) off his waist. He started at 15 st 2 lbs (96.2 kg) and his waist measured 42 ins (107 cm). He is fifty years old and 5 ft 11 ins (1.79 m) tall. Today, 14 May 1991, he is 14 st 2 lbs (89.8 kg) and his waist is 37 ins (94 cm)! He ideally wants to be 12 st 7 lbs/13 st (79.4/82.5 kg), which looks like being reality soon.

I am thirty-eight years old, 5 ft 1 in (1.55 m), and when I dared to get on the scales, as they shot up to 11 st 7 lbs (70.3 kg) and crept up, I jumped off! *Horrified.* At this moment I am just under 10 st 7 lbs (66.7 kg), and have lost 2–3 ins (5–8 cm) from my waist, 2 ins (5 cm) from my hips and 1 in (2.5 cm) from my thighs and above my knees. My bust has not altered, although my back is firmer, and the feeling is terrific! I keep going into the bedroom to have "try-ons" of clothes that were too tight only one month ago, which now fit or are too big! I bought a skirt about a month ago. I tried it on for work yesterday, 13 May 1991, and it nearly fell to the ground. The results are so amazing! Also, I have now got cheekbones (as my face is square, these soon disappear when I put weight on) and my hip-bones are reappearing. I am small-boned, shoe size 3–4, so I want to be 8 st/8 st 7 lbs (50.8/53.9 kg) and I really intend reaching this weight.

As I work in a bakery, I feel even more confident as the smell of fresh bread is forever in my office and my willpower has got stronger. I only need to think of my clothes – this is incentive enough to carry on.

As our class ends this week, Pat and I have resolved to play your video at least three times a week to ensure we keep ourselves toned up. As the results are so noticeable, this is our incentive and it helps the will power to refuse cakes, biscuits, chocolates, etc. I have also noticed my face seems smoother and healthy-looking now, similar to how it looked years ago! Pat did not weigh as much as me – she was 10 st 2 lbs (64.4 kg), but within one month was down to 9 st 6 lbs (59.9 kg). I think

69

this is great as she has two young boys and still has to buy cakes, biscuits etc. for them, but does not indulge herself at all . . .

So this is another success story which has not ended yet. Fred and I started on 21 April 1991, Pat, one week before us, but we all intend to continue eating like this in the future. We go to Newquay in August for a week, so I hope we can continue the diet then, which I am sure we will be able to do.

We would all like to say a big thank-you for helping us to alter our eating habits and I am passing it on to my workmates who are all seeing for themselves the results.'

One married couple who wished to remain anonymous wrote:

'We must say this is the first time that we have stayed on any diet as long as this without great hardship – we both have 1 stone (6.4 kg) to lose and hope to make it.'

After eight weeks the husband had lost 12 lbs (5.4 kg) whilst his wife had lost 9 lbs (4.1 kg).

I was particularly pleased to receive a letter from a vicar's wife and to hear that she and her husband had been following my diet. (Being a committed Christian myself, I am always particularly delighted to hear from anyone connected with the Church.) Here is what Mrs K., the vicar's wife, said:

'I feel I must write to you about the success we have had on your diet. Both my husband and

I started it the week that the article appeared in the *Sunday Express*. As soon as the book was published we were able to get down to it properly. We have both literally changed shape!

I have lost 12 lbs (5.4 kg), nearly all of it from my hips, 47 ins (119 cm) down to 41 ins (104 cm), and 2 ins (5 cm) from my waist. My husband is 1¼ st (8 kg) lighter and has to wear braces to keep his trousers from falling down.

The best thing about this diet, apart from losing weight in the right places, is that there is no calorie counting as such. Wherever we are we can avoid, or restrict, one type of food, and most of the time it is not apparent that we *are* dieting. I call it the *quiet diet*! Now that we have lost weight so noticeably people are showing interest and I have no doubt that there will be a lot of fat lost in this county this summer.'

Mrs K. lost 1 in (2.5 cm) from her bust, making it 36 ins (91 cm), 2 ins (5 cm) from her waist and 6 ins (15 cm) from her hips. After eight weeks Mrs K. had lost 15 lbs (6.8 kg) whilst the Reverend K. had lost 21 lbs (9.5 kg). Four years later, Mrs K. has reduced her weight by a further 6 lbs (2.7 kg) and the Reverend K. has almost doubled his weight loss to 41 lbs (18.6 kg).

On the subject of the *quiet diet* one lady wrote:

'Amazingly successful. I have a husband who is a big eater and any diet I attempted was a failure since he thought I was starving. This diet I can follow without him even noticing I'm on one.

I lost 7 lbs (3.2 kg) within the first ten days

and then nothing for a week, but have lost steadily but slowly since. I must modify the diet for the next ten days as we have guests and are going away, but I shall be able to cut out almost all fats without anyone being the wiser. I feel marvellous, am able to bend and walk briskly, and the arthritis in my knees is greatly improved. Having achieved my objective to lose a stone (6.4 kg) by Easter, I am now aiming for a weight of 11 st (70 kg), and ultimately 10 st 7 lbs (66.8 kg). I am so grateful to you – the weight loss is gratifying but even better is the loss of inches and the emerging of hips and waist.

I passed your diet on to two friends who didn't quite believe me; they have each lost 8 lbs (3.6 kg) and have happily eaten their words.'

Mrs Beatrice Love wrote that her husband had topped 14 st (89 kg) after Christmas. At 5ft 8ins (1.73 m) and working as a painter and decorator, Mrs Love explained that 'he felt far from well, bloated and uncomfortable. Nothing fitted him and his weight was hampering his climbing and bending.' She continued:

'We both began to follow your diet the day after reading the *Sunday Express* and as soon as your book appeared in the shops I bought it. We've never looked back from then. Bill wants to lose another 5 lbs (2.3 kg) or so, bringing him to 11½ st (73.2 kg), he's now 11 st 12 lbs (75.4 kg). He's regaining his boyish figure. My weight had shot up to 10 st 10 lbs (68.2 kg), I'm 5 ft 4 ins (1.62 m). I'm now 9½ st (60.4 kg) and would like to lose another stone (6.4 kg). I'm thrilled about how the fat has gone from my thighs, waist and hips, and my figure is showing some resemblance to the way it looked in my twenties. In fact we are both feeling younger and healthier and our way of life now will be a fat-free one.'

Veronica Jarvis started the diet on her own but after a fortnight her husband joined her.

'I found it much easier, and even visitors have been surprised how well we eat and have joined the Hip and Thigh Brigade.

PS It's not like being on a diet. We were amazed how easy it was to adapt to.'

Ken Wilkins was one of the few men who actually completed the comments section of the questionnaire himself. He wrote:

'I read your book which my wife had bought. She started the diet, so as moral support I followed her eating routine with her. I thought I wasn't overweight at 11 st 2 lbs (70.9 kg). I was amazed at the loss of weight to 10 st 7 lbs (66.8 kg) and not any ill effects yet! Your book contains good sense for a healthy body.'

Mr Edward Bean wrote:

'I feel I can recommend this diet to anybody. My introduction to the Hip and Thigh Diet came by way of a visit to a friend in London. He had a wife who I always knew as a rotund person. Imagine my astonishment when I saw her after a long parting as a very slim youthful figure. My mind was immediately made up and I started there and then.'

Margaret and Douglas Hirst wrote:

'After hearing and reading such glowing reports of your Hip and Thigh Diet I decided it was exactly what was needed by my husband and me. That was six weeks ago. My husband is now 1 st (6.4 kg) lighter – 15 st to 14 (95 kg to 89 kg), all off the offending bulge in front. I have lost ½ st (3.2 kg) – from 9½ to 9 st (60.5 kg to 57 kg). We thoroughly enjoy your menus and eat them heartily, never feeling hungry between meals – though we still occasionally long for a chocolate.'

In their questionnaire which they completed after writing to me, Mrs Hirst explained that she didn't really need to diet 'though I am thrilled that I have lost my spare tyre!' She only followed the diet because her husband needed to lose weight and it made life easier if they both ate the same meals.

'The meals are so enjoyable and appetizing. I prefer them to the meals we used to eat.'

Mr Hirst explained that he had had heart surgery so a very low-fat diet was ideal for his condition.

'I feel 100% better since I started the diet. You see I used to eat a large packet of indigestion tablets per month. Since starting the diet I haven't eaten one. You have my permission to quote me if you wish.'

74

Mr R.E. lost all his excess weight in eight weeks – a remarkable 21 lbs (9.5 kg). He lost 2½ ins (6 cm) from his chest, 2 ins (5 cm) from his waist and 2½ ins (6 cm) from his hips. Mrs E. lost less weight by comparison, but is quite small-boned taking very small-sized shoes and measuring only 4ft 10 ins (1.47 m) tall. In eleven weeks she reduced her weight by 14 lbs (6.4 kg) to 8 st 2 lbs (51.8 kg). She was amazed at the 4½ ins (11 cm) lost from her hips and over 2 ins (5 cm) from each thigh and commented on how much her tummy had reduced. I had to smile when she wrote:

'My husband tells me that since being on the diet I have stopped snoring – he is delighted!'

5

Eat your way to better health

When a smoker dies of lung cancer, the poor victim
is almost always blamed for his or her own death.
'It's not surprising she met an early grave, she's
smoked forty a day ever since I've known her and
that's thirty years,' and, 'What do you expect, smoking all her life – God rest her soul,' are common
judgements made by those left behind.

Among many other factors, it is probably true that
smoking may be a contributory cause of the disease.
But the point is that lung cancer is *immediately* connected with smoking, in everybody's mind.

On the other hand, if someone dies of a heart
attack it is just accepted that the cause is hereditary –
'He over-exerted himself once too often,' or, most
commonly, it was 'Just bad luck'. We have not yet
been sufficiently educated to realize that the risk of
dying from the greatest killer disease in the Western
world could be drastically reduced if only we took
preventative measures by eating sensibly and looking
after our bodies. The earlier we take these steps the
better for everyone concerned.

One in four deaths in this country is caused by
heart disease. This year over 200,000 people will die
from heart disease; that's Wembley Stadium filled
to capacity twice over! No other condition claims so

many lives – yet how many people really know what risks they run? If you were to ask twenty men or women in the street what they should do to avoid heart disease the majority would say, 'Take more exercise, and eat margarine instead of butter.' We are, in reality, extremely ignorant of the various causes of this greatest killer disease.

Whilst there are many types of heart disease, the most common and the most tragic is the type that causes heart attacks and is called coronary heart disease. Here's how it comes about:

Most of us have seen a heart in one form or another, whether on television or in school or even at the butchers. The human heart is about the size of a fist and is a muscle filled with blood. It contracts about seventy times a minute pumping blood around our body. The heart needs a constant good supply of oxygen which it gets from the bloodstream. However, the heart's own oxygen supply is not taken from the blood which is continually being pumped through it to service the rest of the body, but from separate little arteries which are called coronary arteries. These branch off from the main artery, called the aorta, and then divide into lots of smaller branches which are all over the surface of the heart.

The problems start in early adult life when the walls of these coronary arteries become 'furred up' and narrower. The narrowing is caused by a fatty deposit called atheroma and if it gets too thick and the coronary arteries too narrow, the blood supply to the heart becomes restricted or even blocked. This condition is called 'coronary heart disease'.

The disease has two main forms, angina and heart attack. Angina occurs when the coronary arteries have become narrower very gradually and is only noticed when the heart has to work harder than usual. The symptoms of angina are a heavy cramp-like pain across the chest which can spread to the neck, shoulder, arm and even the jaw. Angina is quite different from a heart attack because it is usually relieved by a short period of rest or relaxation. It can also be relieved or controlled by drugs and, in severe cases, surgery.

On the other hand, a heart attack occurs when there is a sudden and severe blockage in one of the coronary arteries so that the blood supply to part of the heart is actually cut off. The blockage is usually caused by a blood clot forming in an artery already narrowed by fatty atheroma. This is called a coronary thrombosis or just 'a coronary'. In some cases the effects of the blockage can be so severe that the heart stops beating altogether and this is called a cardiac arrest. Unless the heart starts beating again within a few minutes the person will die, and in 50% of all fatal heart attacks the victim dies within thirty minutes.

The pain is a crushing vice-like ache felt in the chest. It can also spread to the neck, arm or jaw and doesn't usually ease off for several hours. Sickness, giddiness and feelings of faintness often accompany the pain.

There are many factors which affect our vulnerability to heart disease. As well as our family history, sex and age, we must also consider how physically active we are, the amount of stress we have to endure, whether or not we smoke, what we eat and, very importantly, whether or not we are overweight.

People who have a family history of heart disease are undoubtedly at greater risk. It is obvious that they should take *particular* care to follow preventative guidelines to reduce their risk to a minimum. There is no doubt that the older we get the greater is the risk of suffering a heart attack. The narrowing of the arteries which can lead to angina and heart attacks tends to increase with age. Men are more at risk from heart disease than women. In fact, a man in his late forties is five times more likely to die of heart disease than a woman of the same age. But it would be a mistake for women to consider themselves reasonably 'safe', because after the menopause a woman loses the protective effect of her hormones and her chances of suffering from heart disease are almost equal to a man's. In recent years there has in fact been an increased incidence of heart disease in women in their thirties and forties.

Apart from age, sex and family history, the other contributory factors are voluntary so the choice really is ours!

Cigarette smoking can double our risk of dying from a heart attack and heavy smokers are even more likely to die young. For instance a man who is over fifty and who smokes over twenty cigarettes a day is *four* times more likely to suffer from heart disease than a non-smoker of the same age. Women smokers are just as much at risk as men and at even greater risk if over the age of thirty-five and on the pill. The answer here must be to give up smoking – as soon as you do, you begin to reduce the risk of a heart attack. And the good news is that you could be almost back to a non-smoker's risk level within a few years. Cutting down or smoking low-tar cigarettes will not protect you against heart disease.

The reason cigarette smoking adversely affects the heart is because the nicotine in tobacco smoke increases the blood pressure. This is because the carbon monoxide content of cigarette smoke cuts down the amount of oxygen in the blood and accordingly the heart has to work harder yet it is getting less oxygen. Smoking also speeds up the 'furring up' of the arteries in the heart. Smoking is bad news from every angle – from being damaging to your health and the health of those around you to being smelly and totally antisocial.

A great deal of heart disease could also be prevented if everyone over the age of thirty-five had their blood pressure checked every few years by their doctor. Blood pressure is the pressure which the heart and arteries apply in order to squeeze the blood around the body. When we are sitting or resting our blood pressure remains at a steady resting level. This level increases depending on our activity and the demand for a surge of blood to be sent where it is needed, for instance to the muscles during exercise or to our brain when under pressure mentally. As soon as we stop exerting ourselves the blood pressure returns to normal again.

Hypertension, or high blood pressure, is when the resting blood pressure is higher than normal. Whilst high blood pressure is rare among young people it is common among those over thirty-five, no doubt caused by following an unhealthy lifestyle – eating too much, consuming too much alcohol, having too much salt in our food, smoking, lack of exercise, and suffering from too much stress. Unfortunately most people have no idea that they have high blood pressure because it doesn't actually *feel* any different. But high blood pressure makes the heart work harder resulting in heart disease. There is also the danger of a stroke which is when a blood clot occurs in the brain and the blood supply is cut off.

The good news is that blood pressure can be helped enormously by reducing your weight to its correct level, by not drinking too much alcohol, by stopping smoking, eating less salt, increasing the amount of exercise and by learning to relax.

Stress and anxiety are often self-inflicted. I believe that every problem can be resolved, and that if it can be approached sensibly and thoughtfully, it can even be turned to advantage. If ignored, stress not only contributes to physical disorders such as heart disease, high blood pressure, ulcers and asthma, it can also lead to a variety of mental illnesses of which insomnia, depression and irritability are just early symptoms. On the other hand, if we are under-stressed we will become lethargic and tired and psychosomatic illnesses could occur. A certain amount of stress, therefore, is an essential part of our everyday life. It keeps us on our toes.

Whilst exercise is regularly advocated as essential to a healthy heart this recommendation is often mis-understood. If an overweight man in his fifties who is a heavy smoker, has a family history of heart disease and is working in a stressful job were to decide to 'get fit' and invite a colleague for a game of squash for the first time in twenty years, he would be doing just about the best he could to give himself a heart attack. His heart just would not be able to cope with the strain. The heart will benefit most from the kind of exercise that builds up stamina – the ability to keep going without gasping for breath. Stamina depends on the efficiency of our muscles and circulation and of course the most important muscle of all is the heart itself.

Regular moderate exercise such as brisk walking is the answer for the gentleman described above. As he becomes fitter he may be able to do more and more, but moderation is the key factor. Playing golf or walking the dog is ideal exercise for anyone and the fresh air will be beneficial too. In order to build stamina something more energetic like swimming, cycling or keeping fit to music can be very beneficial and enjoyable. Regular exercise of this kind improves the balance of fatty substances in the bloodstream, lowers the resting blood pressure level and strengthens the heart muscle. But whatever it is we decide to do, it must be continued in the long term. A mad spurt of extreme physical activity for two weeks a year will do us nothing but harm. It is therefore essential to find a form of activity we enjoy so that we are happy to practise it two or three times a week and continue it for life.

So now to the problem of obesity. Obesity can also increase the risk of heart disease, not in itself but because of the many other conditions it can create, conditions which most certainly *do* contribute to heart disease (high blood pressure and diabetes are the most common). The more overweight you are the more likely you are to get high blood pressure and diabetes. Often members of my slimming classes have been referred to me by their doctors, anxious for their patients to reduce their weight and so help reduce their blood pressure. As soon as they lose weight their blood pressure returns to normal.

Don't forget it is not just ourselves we are putting at risk. If we serve bad-for-you foods at home we affect our own hearts, certainly, but worse still, we are serving the wrong food to our families. We have their hearts in our hands too.

There is little doubt that to have become obese in the first instance we have simply eaten too much of the wrong sorts of foods. In other words, too many fatty and sugary foods which are positively loaded with calories – bread spread with lashings of butter, an abundance of fried foods, cream cakes, biscuits, chocolate, crisps and so on. The types of foods overweight people love.

The fat in our food is not only responsible for the extra inches on our hips. It can also push up our blood cholesterol level. (See pages 93–4 for list of foods high in cholesterol.) Cholesterol is a natural substance in the blood and is found in the animal fats we eat, though the body itself is quite capable of making an adequate supply. If there is a lot of fat in our diet we have a high cholesterol level. This can have the effect of accelerating the build-up of atheroma which in turn eventually leads to heart disease. Therefore the higher the level of cholesterol in the blood the greater the risk of problems with the heart.

There has been so much talk of saturated and unsaturated fats that most people have heard of them. Few, however, actually understand what they are. The difference between the two types is their chemical make-up and whilst I don't want to go into lengthy explanations about the proportions of carbon and hydrogen atoms that determine the types of fatty acids it is important to realize that fat isn't just a single compound but comes in many forms. All fats are made up of fatty acids: some of these are saturated fatty acids (called saturates), the rest are unsaturated and these include a special group called polyunsaturated fatty acids (or polyunsaturates). Different fats have different proportions of various fatty acids. Most are high in saturates but some are high in polyunsaturates.

As far as the heart is concerned saturates are considered the main enemy. If we eat too much food high in saturates it can increase our blood cholesterol level and that in turn increases our risk of heart disease. Saturated fat is to be found mostly in animal products like cream, butter, eggs, offal, and in the fat on meat and poultry. In place of butter or margarine, alternatives such as Flora are recommended as it is high in polyunsaturates.

It would be a mistake to *increase* the consumption of foods high in polyunsaturates in the belief that they will 'do us good'. We must, after all, remember that we can produce sufficient cholesterol within our own bodies and that fats high in polyunsaturates contain the *same* amount of calories as the original saturated products, so they do *not* aid slimming in any way.

So this now leaves us with the view that if we reduce our intake of *all* fat our health will certainly benefit and so will our waistlines. And whilst it is impossible to state categorically that heart disease can be caused by eating too much fat, in recent investigations it was observed that among the groups of people who consumed high amounts of fat the incidence of heart attack was far higher than among those who followed a low-fat diet. It would be easy to conclude from this research that fat can actually cause heart disease but with so many other factors to be taken into consideration it is impossible to make such a simple statement. However, it *is* generally acknowledged that to reduce the consumption of fat in our daily diet will almost certainly reduce the risk of heart disease along with other medical conditions.

So how much fat do we actually need? The average

consumption of fat in the Western world at the present time is about 130 grams (over 4½ ounces) a day per person. This fat includes everything from the obvious fats like butter and oil to those hidden in cakes, biscuits and fried foods. The amount of fat we actually *need* is staggeringly low at 5 grams (less than a quarter of an ounce) per day, providing it contains the right kind of fatty acids. As I do not suggest or recommend that we reduce our intake to such a very low level, we need not concern ourselves that we will eat insufficient quantities to endanger our health. However, it is clear that currently far too much fat is consumed and it is an ideal area in which to make a significant reduction without fear of nutrient deficiency.

So, to sum up, if we want to help ourselves towards a healthy heart and a long and happy life we need to eat a low-fat diet, take regular exercise and stop smoking. If we can reduce our weight to around that of our youth and eat well enough to give us the energy to work and live our lives to the full, we will all benefit. In addition, we will make our GPs very happy!

Many of my readers have written to tell me how much their health has benefited from following my low-fat Hip and Thigh Diet. So, while I am not suggesting that my diet will cure or even help anyone suffering from a particular medical condition, I would like everyone to share the experiences of the many people who have found they feel more healthy, more active – much better in every way – since adopting a low-fat diet.

If you are suffering from any illness or medical condition, it is *always* better to go and see your doctor before you start a diet, to discuss how it will affect you. Mrs Janis Kempson, who wisely took this precaution, wrote:

'I took your *Hip and Thigh Diet* book to my doctors to make sure it was okay for me, as two weeks before they told me *not* to go on a diet yet. My doctor took one look at the book and said, "Yes, it is a very good diet, go ahead."

After having a full hysterectomy and six operations for breast cancer, I was feeling very low, but I'm now feeling better than I've felt for a long time. I know I have more pounds to take off. I'm staying on the diet to see if I can lose some more and I will let you know how I get on. In total, I have lost 30¾ ins (77 cm), which is great. I've had plenty of parties, to do with my husband's job, to go to in the eight weeks but I was careful.'

Now let's see how readers suffering from different conditions have felt while following the diet:

Arthritis

Audrey Bewley wrote:

'I suffer from osteoarthritis in my knees. The pain is much reduced and I can walk more easily through the weight loss. The most important comment I have to make is that the awful indigestion and heartburn have disappeared. I truly love the diet and intend keeping to a low-fat diet for the rest of my life.'

Mrs Dennett wrote:

'The results are superb . . . my arthritis has diminished in my feet and hands.'

One lady whose age fell into the 75–84 age group in the questionnaire told me that she had developed arthritis in her right leg last year, and had gained a lot of weight caused by the enforced immobility.

'I am now able to move about much more easily – thanks to you and your most excellent diet. I am amazed to find that I am never hungry whereas before I was always thinking about my next meal. I shall never return to my old way of eating!'

Another lady wrote:

'I feel marvellous, am able to bend and walk briskly and the arthritis in my knees is greatly improved.'

Mrs E.K. wrote:

'Amazed how quickly flesh fell away. In two months I lost 1½ st (9.5 kg) – this cannot be bad! Have tried calorie *control* and lost 5 lbs (2.3 kg) in a fortnight and then stuck.

The effect on health, too, has been astounding. Neck and upper arm arthritis gone and lower back vastly improved (having had spinal fusion, the most I can hope for.)

My whole outlook on life has vastly improved and I feel younger than my seventy-three years. I have regained that sparkle. Many thanks.'

Mrs Sheila Lungley wrote:

'I attended a BUPA Well Woman Clinic on 3 March and to my horror I was told I was 3 st (19 kg) overweight. The nursing sister told me to buy a copy of your book, which I did that same day, and the next day (4 March) I started your diet. I weighed 12 st 13 lbs (82 kg) and three weeks on I am 12 st (76 kg). Well, I cannot believe it. It's the best diet I have ever been on and believe you me I have tried everything including Cambridge and Slimfast Diets, but I was always hungry. In the past three weeks I haven't felt hungry at all and I don't feel the need to binge any more. Losing a stone in such a short time has amazed me, also the loss of inches: 4 March – 12 st 13 lbs (82 kg) – 38–37–42 ins (97–94–107 cm) – widest part 44 ins (112 cm); 25 March – 12 st – 38–34–39 ins (97–86–99 cm) – widest part 40 ins (102 cm).'

Sheila asked us to send her a questionnaire. After she had followed the diet for eight weeks, Sheila returned it along with the wonderful news that by this time she has lost 1 st 7 lbs (9.5 kg), nothing off her bust, 5 ins (13 cm) off her waist, 4 ins (10 cm) off her hips and 6 ins (16 cm) off her widest part, with 2 ins (5 cm) from each thigh and each knee. She also commented:

'As you can see I have had great success over the past eight weeks and I am continuing to keep to the diet until I reach at least 10 st (63.5 kg). I had severe arthritis in both arms, but since I embarked on this diet it has virtually disappeared. I am only forty-six and I had visions of being crippled with it by the time I was fifty years old. I can only thank you for such a wonderful new way of eating. I don't even feel as if I am on a diet, although my weight loss now is averaging 2 lbs (0.9 kg) a week. I get a thrill every week to find I am still losing, it's encouraging me to carry on and to try and lose the same amount again in the coming weeks. I have also regained my confidence once more and my husband thinks I'm a lot happier, which I am.'

Mrs S.W. lost 28 lbs (12.7 kg) in fourteen weeks and with it a staggering 11 ins (28 cm) from her hips! She lost only 1½ ins (4 cm) from her bust, 4 ins (10 cm) from her waist and 5 ins (12.7 cm) from each thigh.

'We have quite a history of rheumatism and arthritis in our family and before losing the weight on the diet I had several twinges in my hips. But with less weight to carry around I have had no more problems.'

Then I received a completed questionnaire from a doctor who had followed the diet and lost 12 lbs (5.4 kg) in seven weeks. This is what she wrote:

'I am actually a doctor interested in, though not dealing in or treating, nutritional problems. I am involved, voluntarily, in Arthritis Care and have recommended this diet to several of our members. Excess weight aggravates arthritis, and yet forced inactivity, because of disability, promotes weight gain.

It remains to be seen how our members benefit

from this regime – certainly they cannot take others (the very low calorie branded powder products) as they can interfere with their drug treatments.

I intend to stick with the diet and lose more, but am satisfied with the steady loss.'

Backache

There are a high number of causes, from poor posture to sciatica, which can give rise to backache. Anyone who has a known back problem, or has undergone surgery on their spine, will be advised to keep their weight down.

I received the following comment on the questionnaire returned by Julie Taylor in Australia:

'I think the diet is fantastic and I feel really great, much healthier. I suffer no more back problems, which I used to have every morning. I must mention my husband Barry. He's been great. He's helped me a great deal and he's been on it too. He's lost 13 lbs (6 kg). He feels better and cannot believe what you are allowed to eat as he likes his food . . .!'

Blood pressure

It is generally accepted that overweight and bad eating habits can contribute to high blood pressure and by reducing weight and amending our diet the problem can be helped greatly. These are some of the comments I received from readers of the Hip and Thigh Diet:

On page 71 we read about the successful weight-loss campaign of Mrs K. and her husband, the Reverend K. After eight weeks Mrs K. had lost 15 lbs (6.8 kg), whilst the Reverend K. had lost 21 lbs (9.5 kg).

Since returning the original questionnaire, Mrs K. has reduced her weight by a further 6 lbs (2.7 kg) and reports a feeling of general good health and increased activity as a result, whilst her husband had almost doubled his weight loss to 41 lbs (18.6 kg) and has now stopped taking his medication for high blood pressure.

Mrs E.D.S. wrote:

'I am convinced that having red meat only twice a week has reduced my blood pressure. The last count was the lowest for nine years.'

Mrs E.B., having lost 2 st (12.7 kg), wrote:

'My doctor is especially pleased as my high blood pressure has gone down five points.'

Mr and Mrs C. wrote to say how delighted they were that both their blood pressure and cholesterol levels had reduced. Mrs C. added:

'I have had high blood pressure since the start of my change of life, also asthma and hot flushes. My blood pressure has gone down from 140/90 to 130/85 since starting the diet; for my asthma I only need to take my spray 2–3 times a week; and as for my hot flushes, I am having a good night's sleep, which my husband is more than pleased about. My husband has lost 10 lbs (4.5 kg) and feels so much better and has a lot more energy.'

Among the many thousands of letters I have received since the *Hip and Thigh Diet* has been published, this one, which came in June 1991, will always rank as one of the most special:

'Dear Rosemary,

It would be understandable that you receive thousands of thank-you notes, but allow a fellow-Christian to add another from a Christian perspective. My wife, Pauline (who is the world's number 1 "honey"), some years ago developed extremely bad blood pressure, having to be on severe medication for the rest of her life. Then sugar diabetes appeared to make her life difficult. Finally, gallstones brought terrible bouts of pain, often for hours.

Consequently, Pauline went on your Hip and Thigh Diet, though at first she did not realize it. By this I mean she cut out all fats and moved more to a vegetable/salad base to help treat the gall condition. Then Pauline found your book and applied its principles and dietary advice.

The end of it was she had lost *4½ st* (28.6 kg) and feels great. We strongly feel that by God's grace and the diet the following has happened: Pauline now has *no* trace of the blood pressure problem, *or* sugar diabetes and the gallstone problem is under control by diet. Often Pauline has said, "I'd like to send Rosemary Conley a 'before' and an 'after' photo", and seeing I had this opportunity, I am conveying her thanks.

I leave today for USA for another five weeks

of ministry after being in the UK for five weeks. Then home to the most wonderful woman in the world.

From Pauline I say, "thank you". From one Christian to another, "thank you". I loved Pauline deeply before she lost the weight, but her feelings about herself, her enjoyment with her new "image", has caused literally scores of other pastors' wives to ask "how did you do it?" She faithfully directs them to your book. She's a treasure.

Respectfully and gracefully yours,
Reverend Ivan Herald, Australia.'

As I was away in Australia on tour two months later, I was able to take the opportunity of accepting a dinner invitation from Ivan and Pauline. I will never forget that evening. They very kindly took me to a revolving restaurant at the top of a tall tower overlooking Sydney Harbour. It was a privilege to spend time with these very special people.

Cholesterol

Notes to cholesterol patients
The low-fat diet described in this book will certainly help those who suffer from high cholesterol, but some foods whilst low in fat are actually very high in cholesterol and anyone who has a high-cholesterol problem should avoid the following foods:

Eggs, egg dishes, Scotch eggs
Offal: Brain, heart, kidney, liver, sweetbread, tongue, liver sausage, pâté
Duck, dark meat of chicken or turkey, steak and kidney pie, lamb, pork, salami

Fish roe, kedgeree, whiting, sardines, mackerel,
  taramasalata
Butter, margarine, cream, cheese, suet
Pastry, cakes, biscuits, buns
Seafood including crab, lobster, prawns, scampi,
  shrimps, mussels, whelks, winkles
Nuts including peanuts, cashews
Mayonnaise, salad cream
Chocolate, crisps
Coconut and coconut oil
Lemon curd

Coeliac disease

This is a digestive disorder requiring the patient to
adhere strictly to a gluten-free diet.

Maureen Watkins wrote to me reporting the beneficial effects of the Hip and Thigh Diet on her shape,
though of course there would have been many foods
suggested in the diet that Maureen would have had
to avoid.

'I am a coeliac on a gluten-free diet. Before
being diagnosed two years ago my tummy was
distended (one of the symptoms). On the gluten-
free diet I put on weight and went up two dress
sizes. The consultant told me I would put on weight
and didn't hold out much hope of my tummy
reducing.

Though the tummy is still more prominent
than I like, there is much less of it and I can pull
it in to look better.

I saw my consultant after four weeks on your
diet, told him I was losing 2 lbs (0.9 kg) a week

and he said it was fine to continue, as eating less fat would be good for me.

I certainly feel and look much better. I have also noticed that my wrists and fingers have slimmed down.

I am continuing with the diet.'

Constipation

Because the diet contains so much natural fibre in the form of fruit, vegetables, cereals and wholemeal bread, I felt confident that it would help many who suffered from constipation. I asked about this in my questionnaire and 86% said they experienced no problems with constipation whilst on the diet. Indeed, many said the diet had definitely helped them to become regular after a history of constipation.

Diabetes

Whilst I would never suggest that the Complete Hip and Thigh Diet is specifically suitable for diabetics, it does contain generous portions of carbohydrates and could easily be adapted to help this condition. I received the following letter from Claire Davison:

'Three weeks ago I met a patient at the Diabetes Outpatients Department of my local hospital where we were waiting to see the consultant. At 16½ st (104.8 kg), with diabetes, an under-active thyroid and very high cholesterol levels, I was a mess. The consultant told me "diet or die". He is known for his plain speaking. The lady I met lent me a copy of your *Hip and Thigh*

Diet. She had lost 3 st (19 kg) in three and half months. I have since bought my own copy and persuaded several others to do so . . .

I have lost a stone (6.35 kg)! And have never in all my fat life (I was 11 st 1 lb [70.3 kg] at ten years old) eaten so much food, or felt so well, or had so much energy. I feel like a teenager again (I'm fifty-six years old) . . . I can't tell you how wonderful it feels to enjoy what I eat. I'm allergic to food colourings and even the local hospital can't come up with colour-free, fat-free and sugar-free diets. I find the portions large, but I'm eating until I'm satisfied at every meal and not missing any meals because I've gained weight.

You are my saviour, I hope to live a long life on your diet. I won't go back to my old habits – I can't face my favourite breakfast of a bacon roll after only three weeks! Butter has lost its taste for me . . . I see the consultant again today and hopefully my sugar and cholesterol levels will be reduced. I'm confident they will.'

Claire then added:

'My diabetic consultant is really pleased with my rapid progress in lowering my very high sugar level and my cholesterol level by over 50% in four weeks.'

Eating disorders

Very often, the delicate subject of 'Eating disorders' arises when I am being interviewed about my diets. Eating disorders, generally speaking, fall into two categories:

Anorexia nervosa, in which the subjects see themselves as larger than they are in reality and avoid food in a desperate attempt to reduce their weight still further. Even when they weigh as little as 5 st (31.7 kg) they consider themselves to be overweight. It is a mental disorder.

Bulimia nervosa, on the other hand, is a condition where the subjects binge and then vomit to remove the food and therefore prevent it depositing fat on the body. Unfortunately, along with the possible weight gain as a result of over-eating, they deprive their body of essential nutrients and deterioration of their teeth is caused by the acidic nature of the bile that is regurgitated.

Both conditions are very serious and certainly anorexia nervosa can lead to death. I always take great pains to dismiss any suggestions of dieting to young girls (these conditions are more prevalent in teenage girls) and emphasize that sensible eating habits are a much safer way of producing a healthy and attractive body. If this low-fat eating plan is combined with plenty of regular exercise the body can remain beautiful into mature years.

I have received several letters from girls who have cured both anorexia and bulimia by following my low-fat diet.

Miss C.W. wrote the following letter:

'I would like to say an enormous "thank-you" for your wonderful diet and to highlight yet another beneficial aspect – in addition to those highlighted in your book.

I am a twenty-two-year-old student (having

lived away from home for more than two years)
who has battled with bulimia nervosa for over seven
years and now finally feel that I've won!

Since following your diet, I have lost nearly
14 lbs (6.3 kg) in five weeks, going from 10 st 1 lb
(64 kg) to 9 st 2 lbs (58 kg), whilst only losing
inches in the "right places". I am now able to eat
virtually as much as I want (I find it impossible to
eat *all* that is recommended anyway) and know
that I need never feel guilty afterwards, thus ending
the cycle of binge–purge–binge etc.

I have recommended your diet to all my friends
and strongly oppose their use of any other means of
weight loss – since the Hip and Thigh Diet retrains
eating habits as well as enabling weight loss.

Thanks to your diet, I feel like a new, energetic,
lively person and can finally begin to come to
terms with and like myself.'

Fiona Cameron from Kent wrote to me in July 1989:

'I am a trained nurse and I've always had a
weight problem. My hips and thighs have always
been bulky, making me feel uncomfortable in
trousers/tight jeans.

I am twenty-three and for the past three years
I have been piling on the pounds without realizing
it, until I finally took a good look at myself –
weighing in at 12 st 3 lbs (77.5 kg) at 5ft 4 ins
(1.63 m).

As a nurse I knew it was unhealthy to be so
overweight and I felt extremely unhappy with
what I had become. I knew I had an eating problem
when I secretly started to buy sweets from several
different shops and to ensure the empty wrappers

were well hidden from my boyfriend. Then I started to make myself vomit and knew my problem was serious.

I had always been an erratic bingey eater and was forever on a diet without losing weight due to bingeing/starving/vomiting. I would always be "starting the diet tomorrow" and if I ate one thing "out of order" the diet would collapse and I would eat everything in sight until I could hardly move.

My boyfriend knew nothing of these habits and the first move was to tell him, which relieved me (actually to admit to someone how unhappy I was with these eating habits). Just after Christmas we decided to get married, so I had till June to diet. I was already feeling depressed about having to lose weight and I hadn't heard of your diet.

Then I bought your book. I was most sceptical when reading all the letters, thinking it must be "fixed". My boyfriend commented that surely I couldn't lose weight eating so much food! I started on 10 April and by 24 June (my wedding day) I had lost 21 lbs (9.5 kg), all from areas usually unshiftable! I couldn't believe how healthy I felt. I no longer craved sweet stuff, no longer felt the necessity to binge, and have only cheated twice, and I mean one chocolate *not* the whole box as before.

As a nurse I cannot think of a healthier diet to follow and can see no disadvantages in the diet. I feel fully satisifed, appetite-wise, and have lost weight easily despite having bread and rice every day. I looked my slimmest ever on my wedding day and thoroughly enjoyed my holiday. I actually ate what I liked without feeling devastated, knowing the diet was at hand. I have never in my life looking forward to starting a diet, but by the end of my holiday I couldn't wait to get back on it so that I could maintain my slimmer figure. On other diets I have put all the weight back on and more.

I used to struggle into a size 14, but now I have a wardrobe full of new clothes – size 10/12. I've lost 4 ins (10 cm) all over and my friends cannot believe it. They've all bought your book! I feel so glad that I've finally found something that works and am not confined to a life of bingeing/ vomiting etc. I can now go out for the odd meal without suffering from the binge factor just because I had a dessert.

I have recommended your diet to various patients as I don't see how anyone can fail to benefit from a low-fat diet. I feel I owe you so much and would love to meet you because this diet has changed my life.

So a big thank-you for such a brilliant diet. I feel fantastic.'

As I was preparing to rewrite the first edition of this book I asked Fiona if she would complete a questionnaire. Her vital statistics, one year on, are an enviable 34–25–34 ins (86–64–86 cm). She commented that it was the 'no calorie counting' and the fact that she could eat so much more than on most diets that were the main reasons for her success and healthier lifestyle. In the comments section she wrote:

'What I like about this diet is that it contains "real food" rather than fluid meals etc., and there is a wide variety – plus it works! The weight does come off the "difficult to shift areas".'

Epilepsy

One lady who prefers to remain anonymous, wrote:

'From the age of seven I have suffered from epilepsy. When I was eleven I started my periods and I had a fit while menstruating. The following week I had another fit. My grandmother took me to the doctors, but they said there was nothing they could do about it. At twenty-six I married a man who had cared for epileptics in a home and he understood all the problems I was having. Sometimes, I would go six months without being poorly, but that was because I spent a few days in bed. Last year I found some of my clothes were too tight around the waist, so first of all I bought your *Inch Loss Plan* video, then my husband bought me your *Hip and Thigh Diet* book, plus *Whole Body Programme* video. I exercised every day to your workouts even when I was on my periods. I am thirty-eight years old and it was been eleven months since I had a fit. Thank you, Rosemary, for your workouts – I think you have helped me more than the doctors ever did.'

Gallstones

As I explained at the beginning of this book, it was due to my own gallstones that this diet was discovered. After my first book about the Hip and Thigh Diet was published I received many letters from fellow sufferers who had avoided major surgery by following a very low-fat diet and who, like me, had enjoyed the side effect of reduced inches on their hips and thighs.

Needless to say there were lots of people who were suffering with gallstones, and awaiting surgery, who were delighted when my *Hip and Thigh Diet* book was published. It gave them a 'handbook of how to avoid fat' – the very food that causes the gall bladder to work and to disturb your gallstones if you have the misfortune to have them.

Here are three extracts from the many letters I received from gallstone sufferers. I received the first, a heart-warming one about Mr T., from his wife:

'My husband (unfortunately now seventy years of age) has suffered for a number of years through inoperable gallstones due to thrombosis and having continually to take warfarin. Last Christmas, because for years he had been unable to eat a decent meal, due also to a hiatus hernia, he decided life was only a mere existence and didn't want to be bothered with anything.

However, having myself attended a local slimming class where they used your low-fat diet I begged my husband to try it. This was a man who had been brought up on a farm, plenty of fat, etc., and who absolutely refused to eat wholemeal bread, cereals or anything of a like nature. What a difference now! Come 17 January he agreed "yes", he would try anything, and after a few days he was able to eat three meals a day and was not regurgitating. In three months he has lost approximately 3½ st (22.2 kg) and now weighs 13½ st (85.7 kg). As you say, it is easy to lose weight, but it is harder to keep it off. Well, he has done just that and he looks and feels wonderful and certainly belies his years and is at least 5 ins (13 cm) less around his waist than before.

He has been under the watchful eye of his surgeon at the local Royal Infirmary for many years, because due to his size, at one time he was afraid he was filling up with water and to help with the constant sickness had each day to take three tablets, which he discontinued on 1 March, with his doctor's approval, of course.

Yesterday morning the surgeon was so pleased with him he said, "You are absolutely wonderful to have done this on your own," and promptly discharged him, saying my husband need no longer come to his department at the hospital. My husband was quick to correct him, saying, "The thanks were entirely due to Rosemary Conley and her healthy eating plan."

"Surely then," said the surgeon, "this is worth a letter of thanks," hence prompting me to write to you immediately.

We neither of us know how to thank you for this help and making our lives worth living again.

I must apologize for going on at length and in passing would say that my only adverse comment is due to having to re-clothe this healthy man of mine.'

Needless to say, Mrs S.T.'s letter brought a lump to my throat.

Mrs Brenchley wrote:

'I am a sixty-two-year-old diabetic with several other health problems and have now had a rather large gallstone diagnosed. They are *very* reluctant to operate, although I have had very severe attacks during the last two years (they only give me a 50–50 chance of success) and I have had to 'learn to live with it'. Your book has helped me to do just that. Since buying it, I have enjoyed the best health I've had for years, as I now know exactly what foods to avoid and am still able to keep up my quota of carbohydrates for the Insulin. I have begun to lose weight very slowly *but* steadily. I showed the book to my doctor, telling her what I was doing – and she agreed that she has seen a great improvement in me. So, I for one am a very satisfied customer.'

Mrs Joyce Williams wrote:

'I started following your diet as soon as I was able to obtain a copy of your book. My reason was to avoid surgery for gallstones – I am seeing a surgeon in three weeks' time – and so far the pain has gone, and so has the excess fat exactly where you said it would! I would like to know if you get any pain now and whether the stones disappear or pass through, or whether they lie quietly waiting for the next indiscretion with food.

I am not looking forward to meeting the surgeon because I imagine he will not be pleased with me when I refuse any surgery offered.'

I replied explaining that fortunately I had not experienced any further pain since changing from a very high-fat to a very low-fat regime, despite the occasional 'indiscretion'. I sent Joyce a questionnaire, and when she replied she wrote:

'My gallstone problem has seemingly disappeared. The weight loss has been a bonus!

I see the surgeon on 11 April and intend to show him your book and to tell him of my improvement. I only had one "bad" episode – nothing like yours – in November, and have waited until April for my appointment! If I elected to have an operation I suppose it could well be a few years before my turn came. I will never again budge from this diet.'

I hope Joyce's gallstones have continued to give her no more trouble but I must point out that an illness is never the same for any two people. I have no doubt that for many my low-fat diet can help enormously in the relief of pain caused by gallstones. I would *never* suggest that you go against the advice of your doctor or surgeon; but there is, I believe, no harm in asking first to try all other avenues to avoid surgery. If this fails, at least you will feel satisfied that you've done what you can. And, five years on, there have been huge advances in surgery for this condition and sufferers are now able to enjoy the luxury of having their gall bladders and gallstones removed by microsurgery. The patient is now in hospital for only twenty-four hours instead of two weeks and the unsightly 14 in (36 cm) scar across the abdomen is avoided. In its place are four minute incisions, which disappear within three weeks of the operation having taken place. This operation is available on the National Health and patients may now return to work within a week rather than, as previously, after an eight-week recovery period.

Heart disease

Heart disease is the biggest killer in the Western world. It can be caused by a combination of many factors. If it runs in the family, if you are a male, you smoke, are overweight and have a stressful life, take very little exercise and eat a lot of fatty food – watch out! I don't wish to alarm you, but these are the facts; and we can do *so* much to help ourselves. Women are also at risk, particularly after the menopause when the protective hormones diminish.

However, never has help been so available to those who are most at risk. The whole medical profession is keen to encourage prevention of heart disease which, for most, *is* avoidable. And it's never too late to start.

Mrs Marsh wrote to me about her husband who had decided to use my Hip and Thigh Diet to help stave off a likely heart attack:

'We used the book not just to lose weight but for medical reasons – my husband *had* to go on a fat- and cholesterol-free diet. He had been told that, with his family history and his high blood fat count, he would have a heart attack within five years – probably fatal. He is forty-three. We were given a diet sheet. Your book made things much easier.

He went for follow-up tests in February – three months after sticking very strictly to the diet.

His blood fat count is down by 30% and the doctor is very pleased and told him to stick to whatever he is doing, and wishes everyone would do the same. His chances of a fatal heart attack have been cut drastically.

The side effects are: we are all, two daughters and ourselves, on a very healthy diet and I have a lean, trim husband again. From us you deserve a *thank-you*.'

On the questionnaire which Mrs Marsh completed on behalf of her husband, she added:

'The diet is a permanent feature of this household, but because of its excellent success rate, when we do have a meal out, we can relax a little and though we do not binge as such, the occasional "wrong" foods are acceptable. Where there has been weight loss we did not take measurements as that was not the *reason* for the diet, but a happy side effect.'

Douglas Hirst, another heart patient, whose letter appeared on page 74, wrote this on his questionnaire:

'I shall still carry on with this diet because I want to try and reach 13 st (82.7 kg). I have had heart surgery and this fat-free diet is so good for my condition. I feel 100% better since I started it.'

Hiatus hernia

A hiatus hernia is a most unpleasant condition which has the effect of allowing food that has been eaten to be regurgitated, and constant belching is experienced by sufferers.

Mrs K. Hayman wrote on her questionnaire:

'I have had quite a lot of trouble with a hiatus hernia for some years. Since going on this diet, I am so much better; no coughing or sickness and I have been able to cut down on the tablets I have to take after meals. It is a wonderful feeling to know I can go anywhere without coughing and worrying about other people.

I thought you would like to see the *do's* and *don'ts* of having an hiatus hernia, and how your diet helps so much.'

Mrs Hayman enclosed a useful list of *do's* and *don'ts* for hiatus hernia sufferers in the hope that they may help other people:

Do's	*Don'ts*
Eat little and often (about 2-hourly).	Eat and drink at same meal.
All liquids including soup should be taken not less than 1 hour before or after solid food.	Eat more than 2 courses at any time.
Chew your food very thoroughly.	Drink anything that is too hot or ice cold.
Peel fruit and tomatoes as the skin is indigestible.	Drink normal tea or coffee as it creates acid.
Drink fruit juices, herb tea, or China tea.	Take white sugar, white bread or white rice.
	Bend forward when lifting or picking up anything, but bend the knees as you lift.

Sweeten with honey or natural brown sugar.

Try to avoid coughing – it can enlarge the hernia.

Try to sleep on high propped-up pillows at night.

Never stretch your arms upwards and avoid wearing restrictive clothing.

Mrs B.R. followed my diet and wrote:

'Having suffered quite severely from a hiatus hernia since 1980 I find the need for less medication than for many years . . . so nice to be free from the dreadful chest pain I had at times, bringing me to many tears.'

I received a lovely letter from May Tapp. With her permission I am quoting it all:

'I would like to say thank you for your book – *Hip and Thigh Diet*. I have followed it to the letter for nearly four months and have lost almost 2 st (12.7 kg) in weight, and all from the right places. The biggest bonus, however, is in how much better I feel. I have angina, a hiatus hernia and a few more problems. The hernia had got completely out of control and I was never free from pain, but almost from the first day of this diet it improved and kept on improving till it doesn't bother me at all now. This I can only describe as a miracle. After eight weeks, I went over to the maintenance diet but found I still wasn't happy with more fat so had a word with my doctor. He said: "Don't worry about having more fat. You are obviously 100% better so stay with it and just increase bread, vegetables and fruit.''

I am seventy this year and feel better now than for a few years past. I recommend the diet to everyone who's interested, but they have to buy their own book. I wouldn't part with mine for anything.

Everything you claimed for it has been *true* in my case and I can't thank you enough for it.

Wishing you every success in the future.'

Indigestion

It was staggering to hear how many people had previously suffered from indigestion and heartburn, but who had found the symptoms disappear after following my diet. Here are just a small sample of the letters I received on this subject.

Elizabeth Hainworth wrote:

'Towards the end of last year I began to suffer from heartburn after every meal. The article about your diet appeared in the New Year, and I played around with it to start with, but after a binge on the cheese (my weakness) which brought on an attack of heartburn, I paid a visit to the doctor. He informed me I was overweight (1 st [6.4 kg]). Your diet was talked about and after that I stuck to it rigidly. Providing I watch the fat content on products the heartburn has virtually disappeared.'

Elizabeth lost 1 st 2 lbs (7.3 kg) in the following eight weeks.

Veronica Jarvis explained that she had been plagued by heartburn for the past two years, 'but not a sign of it these past eight weeks', she said. And Carol Howes wrote on her questionnaire:

'I have dieted in the past, usually losing a pound or two (0.5 to 1 kg) then gaining three or four pounds (1 to 2 kg) and so my weight has steadily increased over the last eighteen years. I accepted the fact that I would just keep getting larger with age – albeit unhappily – and that, short of starvation, I would never be slim again.

My husband read of the Hip and Thigh Diet in the *Sunday Express* and said, "Here's a diet you can do." I was amazed, as this was the first time he'd openly admitted to me that he thought I was fat. "I couldn't do that," I said. "All that fruit would give me the runs!" However, I read it more closely and decided to give it a try. A previous diet with salads and fruit had upset my stomach so I was a little wary at first. One of my favourite fruits is an orange, but I just couldn't eat a whole one without trouble afterwards. This time I thought I'd give one a try and to my delight suffered no ill effects whatsoever and have eaten one a day ever since. The same goes for salads and other fruits – my stomach has never been so "settled".

The other wonderful effect is that I've had no inclination to eat sweets, cakes or chocolates and haven't binged for nearly three months. The past few weeks I've even bought chocolate and chocolate biscuits for the family and can sit and watch them being eaten without any desire for them myself – magic. I am so delighted with the smaller me, and have recommended the diet to

111

family and friends – wishing I had shares in your publishers. Hubby seems quite chuffed too!

I intend to maintain this eating regime and stay slim.'

Migraine

I can't begin to think how absolutely dreadful it must be to suffer from migraine. I grumble if I get a normal headache! I was aware of the benefits of the diet to migraine sufferers because Di Driver, one of my most successful followers of the diet in its original trial stage, was completely cured from this devastating condition after following the diet. I later learned of many more – both men and women. I was therefore not surprised when I began receiving more letters telling me of others' successes in this direction.

Mrs P. Crisp wrote:

'I have suffered cruelly from migraine since 1974 when my husband died, and I know chocolate, hard cheese, oranges and sometimes even wholemeal bread will bring on an attack, but since I went on your diet the attacks have virtually ceased. My dear mother suffered from this all her life but she adored fat on meat, bread, dripping and roast potatoes, and pre-war no one gave a thought to the idea that diet could help her. My doctor is delighted as it has meant far fewer tablets. This morning I had a try-on of summer skirts and slacks and my spirits have soared as my weight has gone down.'

Mrs Crisp, who is 5 ft 2 ins tall (1.57 m) and seventy years old, lost 16 lbs (7.3 kg) in ten weeks on the Hip and Thigh Diet and now weighs 9 st 8 lbs (61 kg).

Linda Goldsmith wrote:

'I am truly amazed by the results and it was so easy! Also my "sick" lethargic headaches seem to have disappeared almost completely. I can only put that down to not eating cream and rich food any more (very difficult as I am a hotelier by trade). I feel much better. My mother was so impressed at the way I look, she has also bought the book and started the diet.'

It's not surprising Linda's mother is impressed – Linda's vital statistics now read 33–26–36 ins (84–66–91 cm). She lost just 1 in (2.5 cm) from her bust, an amazing 4 ins (10 cm) from her waist and a total of 4 ins (10 cm) from her hips and widest part.

I believe the reason for the alleviation of migraine symptoms is that only small amounts of dairy products are allowed in the diet. Also, of course, no chocolate is allowed and this is recognized as a 'baddie' for migraine sufferers.

Pre-menstrual tension

Pre-menstrual tension (PMT) is frequently discussed in the media as it affects so very many women. I have absolutely no idea why my diet should help this condition, but I received several letters in which slimmers explained how their general health and well-being had improved significantly. The first hint was when I received the following letter from Barbara Jones:

'I have now been following your diet for three weeks and so far have lost 13 lbs (5.9 kg) in weight. I have followed many diets over the last ten years. Never have I lost so much so easily and quickly – I normally lose 1–1½ lbs (approx. 0.5 kg) per week. I have found the diet easy to follow and have never felt hungry. I have also been doing the exercises in your book, working out 2–3 times per week and playing squash. I have made some minor adjustments to the recipes shown, as I do not eat very much meat – only white turkey/chicken breast about twice a week. However, I find I can make very tasty meals with chick peas, kidney beans, etc.

As I have kept accurate measurements since Day 1, I should like to take part in your survey and complete the questionnaire.

I would also add that I feel very well following this diet and, as an added bonus, have not suffered from PMT this month, as I normally do.'

I sent Barbara a questionnaire which she returned after following the diet for eight weeks. By then she had lost 24 lbs (10.9 kg) and had reduced her inches magnificently: 3 ins (7.5 cm) off bust and waist, 4 ins (10 cm) from hips and widest part, and 2½ ins (6 cm) from each thigh. She added that her PMT symptoms had disappeared, 'and I feel great', she wrote.

Mrs Aileen Charley lost 18 lbs in eight weeks and ½ in from her bust, 2½ ins (6 cm) from her waist, 2 ins (5 cm) from her hips, 3 ins (7.5 cm) from her widest part, and an inch (2.5 cm) from each of her already slim thighs (now 20 ins [51 cm]). Aileen wrote:

'Since starting this diet I have noticed a great improvement during the week before my periods. My breasts are no longer sore and tender and instead of putting 5–6 lbs (approx 2.5 kg) on during that week I remain the same weight. The spots that used to appear on my face and neck during that week have also gone. I am still breast-feeding my four-year-old daughter so I'm afraid I drink more than ½ pint (250 ml) of semi-skimmed milk a day, but the pounds and inches are still coming off. It's lovely not to be "fat and forty" any more and it's even better being lighter than my fourteen-year-old son who is 6 ins taller than me.'

Pauline Perry wrote telling me that before her monthly period she is usually bad tempered, 'but I feel less ratty than usual'. Pauline lost 19 lbs (8.6 kg) in eight weeks and lost a staggering 8 ins (20 cm) from her widest part.

Mrs B.S. wrote: 'As I mentioned in my letter dated 9 June your diet has helped me with a very painful problem, that of swollen breasts (as part of PMT). I have since been informed by my mother-in-law, who is a GP, that this is one of the few symptoms of PMT that is untreatable. Consequently I hope that many other women that suffer in this way can find relief by cutting out fat from their diet.'

Mrs Jill Davies wrote: 'I have enjoyed this diet and the results are fantastic. Also I used to suffer from

PMT. This has stopped. I liked this diet because the inches went from where I wanted them to go from.'

Jill lost nothing from her 34-in (86 cm) bust, 2½ ins (6 cm) from her waist, 6 ins (15 cm) from her hips, 5 ins (12.7 cm) from her widest part, 4½ ins (11 cm) from each thigh and 3 ins (8 cm) from just above each knee. Her vital statistics are now 34–25½–33 ins (86–65–84 cm).

Pregnancy

Ava Richardson telephoned me shortly after my book was published. She was twenty-six weeks into her pregnancy and wanted to know if she could follow the diet. I recommended that she increase the allowance of milk and protein foods and should show her doctor the diet before commencing. Ava kept me up to date with her progress and condition throughout the remaining weeks. Despite the fact that she suffered from a back problem and had to rest for most of the time, she still managed to lose ¾ in (2 cm) from her hips and widest part, and over 1 in (2.5 cm) from each of her thighs. She told me that despite the fact that she stopped dieting some weeks before the baby was born, her inch losses were maintained despite the gain in her weight. When I spoke to Ava after Gregory Peter had been born (8 lbs 6 oz [3.8 kg]) she said she felt wonderful and was now back on the diet to reduce her weight still further.

NB *Always* check with your doctor first before embarking on any diet during pregnancy.

Underactive thyroid

A nurse wrote to me explaining that she suffered from an underactive thyroid 'so everything was against me'. She continued:

'I would like to thank you for the diet which I am following with no trouble and seeing results already. It is marvellous.'

Mrs Pamela W. wrote to me as follows:

'I am sixty-eight years of age – lost my husband eighteen months ago – have four children and nine grandchildren. With the shock of my husband's death, very suddenly I put on weight to 15 st 5 lbs (97.5 kg). My doctor discovered I had an underactive thyroid, but in spite of that she said she still wanted the weight off. I had arthritis in one hip and to walk a mile was an effort. My doctor recommended your book and is delighted with the result . . .

In twelve weeks I have lost 2 st 3 lbs (14 kg) and with it 6½ ins (17 cm) from my bust, 8 ins (20 cm) from my waist, 5 ins (13 cm) from my hips and 8 ins (20 cm) from my widest part; 4 ins (10 cm) have gone from the tops of my thighs and 3 ins (8 cm) from above the knees.

I went on holiday to Majorca and for the first time in thirty years I put on a bathing costume and shorts and found I swam automatically. "Grandma swimming," was the cry. I danced every night from 8.00 p.m. until 12.00 midnight.

Luckily I ate fruit, melon and continental breakfast and did not gain or lose a pound and I did occasionally have a piece of gâteau or ice cream and fruit. Now I am back on the diet again and hope to get off another half stone. I never feel hungry, but feel so much better in health and energy. My doctor says she tells everyone about me at her clinic and when she gets a few ladies together she wants me to go and talk to them about how I did it. A male cousin seventy-two years old was impressed and has gone on it and has lost 7 lbs (3.2 kg) in a month . . .

A month ago I was able to get into a model dress which I wore for my daughter's wedding twenty-five years ago. As it has not dated, I wore it to go to church three weeks ago.

How can I thank you for the new lease of life you have given me. You are welcome to use any of my remarks.'

So if you are a sufferer, it is well worth a try. But do check with your doctor first.

6
'This diet changed my life!'

We all know that anyone who has to watch their weight feels much more confident when slim. Our outlook and attitude to life is totally different from how we feel when we are overweight. I would suggest that our mental attitude can change so dramatically for the better that we are able actually to *achieve* more than we ever thought possible. Someone who is overweight often feels 'ugly' and subconsciously doesn't *want* to succeed, preferring to disappear into oblivion, hoping that the world will not notice them. But that same person, having successfully lost all their excess weight, becomes a completely different sort of person – creative, confident, positive. Now that person's *ability* won't have changed, but the *desire* to live life to the full will be dramatically increased.

Among the many letters I received, this new mental attitude became very obvious. Catherine Ann Pike wrote:

'I would just like to take this opportunity to say thank you for writing a marvellous book and that losing 3 st (19.1 kg) has certainly changed my life, making me more confident and very happy.'

Miss Imelda Dwyer wrote:

'The confidence and pride in my appearance cannot really be measured, I have experienced a total change in personality with a positive attitude to life which has improved my work and social life. Once again thanks very much.'

Avril Daley wrote this on her questionnaire:

'My husband has also been on your diet and has lost 10 lbs (4.5 kg). He feels so much better and has a lot more energy. So, I would like to thank you for introducing me to your diet; it has made such a difference to me. I have now started an Office Training Course for the unemployed and am learning to type and use a word processor. It has given me confidence to go back out to work and take a pride in myself once again, instead of sitting at home eating.'

Barbara Simmons wrote:

'On 7 February this year I gave birth to my third girl. I didn't really want another baby, because we couldn't afford one more, and being a bit selfish I didn't want to put my body through another pregnancy and birth, knowing I would be carrying excess fat, far more than usual. But I couldn't wait to have her and she is much loved and adored by all of us. After a month I looked in the mirror at my naked body and burst into tears. I couldn't believe how bad I looked. I am only twenty-five years old and looked like I had a body of a fifty-year-old who'd never exercised. So, for my depression, I ate a lot. My husband is very understanding, but he made me worse, because he is 6 foot (1.82 m) of pure muscle. So on 17 April I made him get me all the things I needed to diet. I put my measurements in your book. Just over 9 st (57.2 kg) [I haven't got any scales].

Bust: 35 ins (89 cm)
Waist: 30 ins (76 cm)
Hips and widest part: 36 ins (91 cm)
Thighs: 21 ins (53 cm)
Knees: Left 14¼ ins (37 cm), Right 14 ins (36 cm)
Arms: 11½ ins (29 çm)

It was the inch loss that amazed me – it just fell off. This is my diary of weight loss:

22.4.92
Bust: 34½ ins (87 cm)
Waist: 29 ins (74 cm)
Hips: 35 ins (89 cm)
Widest part: 35½ ins (90 cm)
Thighs: Left 20¼ ins (51 cm), Right 20 ins (51 cm)
Knees: Left 13¾ ins (35 cm), Right 13½ ins (34 cm)
Arms: 10½ ins (26 cm)

4.5.92
Bust: 34 ins (86 cm)
Waist: 28 ins (71 cm)
Hips and widest part: 34¼ ins (87 cm)
Thighs: Left 20 ins (51 cm), Right 19½ ins (50 cm)
Knees: Left 13½ ins (34 cm), Right 13¼ ins (33 cm)
Arms: 10 ins (25 cm)

12.5.92
Bust: 33½ ins (85 cm)
Waist: 27½ ins (70 cm)
Hips and widest part: 34 ins (86 cm)
Thighs: Left and right 19 ins (49 cm)
Knees: Left 13¼ ins (33 cm), Right 13 ins (33 cm)
Arms: 10 ins (25 cm)

And my measurements today (18.5.92) are:
Bust: 33 ins (84 cm)
Waist: 26½ ins (67 cm)
Hips and widest part: 34 ins (86 cm)
Thighs: Left and right 19 ins (49 cm)
Knees: Left and right 13 ins (33 cm)
Arms: 10 ins (25 cm)

My weight is now 8 st 4 lbs (52.6 kg) and I feel fantastic . . . I'm now not on your diet – it's just a way of living for me now, and I'm trying to work my husband into it . . . He took me out on Friday to buy me some clothes. I am now a proud owner of a few size 10 shift-dresses and when I wear them my husband can't keep his hands off me!'

Margaret Venables wrote to me and mentioned that she worked in a voluntary capacity with an international children's organization, meeting a lot of people at all levels. 'Never again will I feel like a stranded whale,' she said – which is exactly how so many overweight people feel when they are in public.

It doesn't help, of course, to have tried to slim for years and to have continually failed. Margaret explained her history of struggling:

'Previously I had been to Weight Watchers – good – expensive – and I soon put back the weight. The specialist sent me to a hospital dietitian and, despite being careful with what I ate, there was no obvious weight loss. My doctor said, "Stop eating," and he gave me tablets to help – again little weight loss and I began to feel at odds with myself.'

Margaret began the Hip and Thigh Diet at the end of January. Her letter continued:

'Yesterday was my third Sunday and I feel great – weight loss so far 5 lbs (2.3 kg). We had our daughter's twenty-first birthday party on Saturday and I still lost weight – 1½ ins (4 cm) from my bust, 1 in (2.5 cm) from my waist – but most important I feel great and your diet has given me back my interest in myself and that is amazing.

No doubt you receive many, many letters – but I just had to write and tell you how I felt.'

I replied to Margaret's letter and asked her to tell me about her progress.

In April, Margaret wrote again and this is what she said:

'I am sending you my "loss" chart for the first eight weeks of my new eating habit.

I find it incredible that I have lost inches even though these eight weeks have included our daughter's twenty-first birthday celebrations, several trips to London for meetings, my own birthday and a parish lunch.

In the past, my efforts to diet have certainly

resulted in the loss of a few pounds and I have watched the scales carefully – but the weight has rapidly returned and I have been back to square one. This new eating habit is so simple – once your palate has adjusted to the new tastes it ceases to be a diet, and I have never felt better.

You mentioned in your letter that you would like to quote me in your next book. If I can help anyone to improve their health, then please feel free to use my comments.'

Margaret's inch losses were totally satisfactory. Her bust had reduced from 38 to 36 ins (96.5 to 91.5 cm), her waist had slimmed by 3½ ins (9 cm), hips by 1½ ins (4 cm) and each thigh had trimmed off 2 ins (5 cm). You can imagine how much more confident Margaret must have felt at the various functions she had attended – particularly her daughter's twenty-first birthday.

Sue Pepi from Australia wrote:

'As you can see from the questionnaire I have lost 29 lbs (13 kg) in eight weeks on your diet (which I call "my way of eating for life") and I intend to lose another 26 lbs (12 kg) to reach my desired weight. I *love* the diet and I *love* the feeling great within myself.'

Sue went on to add within the questionnaire:

'I am so confident of being able to reach my desired weight and, just as importantly, keeping it off – it's reassuring. I feel great and people are commenting on how I am looking great. I must

124

be doing something right. I have so much more confidence and I am so much happier that it flows out of me and people are responding to my positive vibes and attitude. *I love it!*'

Miss J.M., also from Australia, wrote:

'My friends cannot believe that in just a short period of six months I've gone from a fat pimply adolescent 148 lbs (67 kg) to a trim and healthy clear-faced girl 115 lbs (52 kg). They are all very fussy about what they eat so I informed them about your book and they all went and purchased a copy each. Within weeks they had all taken on what seem like a "brand new image", but really it was just a healthy diet. They kept on urging me to write and thank you personally and I have finally got the courage to express my gratitude to you in this letter.'

Another lady who asked to remain anonymous wrote:

'While I was following your diet, and ever since, I have felt so much healthier and, with the renewed confidence in my slimmer self, I feel great! Forgive me for mentioning this but the man in my life has commented on the change in me. He thinks it's his birthday whenever we get together!'

Yes, losing weight and feeling happier about your body certainly does make you feel a lot more contented about yourself when in a close relationship – whether you are simply dancing and not having to worry about your partner feeling folds of fat under your bra as he places his hands on your back, or whether you're making love.

Lorna Cowley wrote that losing weight and finding her confidence had completely revolutionized her life! Lorna's husband was unwell and unable to drive the family car. She had not driven for fifteen years but one day, quite amazingly, she decided to have a go. Living in the country and having a 'family' of animals to feed she discovered she had run low in pet foodstuffs. She took her courage in her hands and managed to drive to the local pet shop. 'I was really nervous,' she said. 'I didn't know where the indicators were and I simply forgot about the seat belt. When I got to the shop I had to ask a farmer to turn the car round for me so that I could drive home!'

Since then she has increased in confidence, drives regularly, even through large towns, and knows how to check the oil, battery, tyres and water. What an achievement!

Lorna wrote so enthusiastically about the positive changes in her life that have made her a totally different sort of person – one she actually feels happy with.

'I am so *very* grateful for your fantastic diet, and really proud of my new trim figure for my age. I have found a super stylist for my hair. When I collected my very expensive new classic suit last week, I was told that if I slimmed down any more – it wouldn't fit me! I felt quite like a model in it!'

What a delightful transformation in attitude.

Margaret Dominey returned her completed questionnaire in July 1991. In the first seven weeks of following the diet she had lost a staggering 30 lbs (13.6 kg) in weight. Thereafter she consistently lost a pound per week so that by the time she was returning her questionnaire her weight was at 10 st 10 lbs (60 kg), which was quite acceptable for her 5 ft 6 ins (1.67 m) frame. The comments section within the questionnaire provided insufficient space for Margaret's message. This is what she wrote:

'For what I wanted to share with you there was no way that I was going to be able to get it into the space for comments. You may use as much, or as little of what I am sharing with you.

My first marriage was at sixteen years old and I had my first son before I was seventeen. When I had him I put on over a stone (6.4 kg) in weight. This was the start of putting on weight and trying to take it off and keep it off. Over the years I've put on and taken off weight, trying so many different ways and trying things I've seen advertised or been told about, etc. By the time I saw your book I was at the "Oh, well, here we go again" stage. Even the thought of something new or different didn't give me any excitement or challenge. Too many years hoping and being disappointed even though I did lose weight. There wasn't one diet about which I could say to myself, or to others, "I have found what I've been looking for", until I read your book. As I read it daily and took it out with me I could see a new challenge and a new excitement each day. This started out as another diet, but I could see what I was buying and eating and I was happy feeling that this was going to be a life-changing experience for me, and that's what I wanted. I share with people of all ages what's happening to me through this book of yours and how it can change their lives as well. Many have seen and remarked on the difference in me and I tell them, "It's not just a diet," and then I start to encourage them to use not only the scales but also the tape measure, etc. . . . how I do not feel hunger and how I lost weight, 30 lbs (13.6 kg) in seven weeks, and many other things. . . . There is so much encouragement I can and do share, and the peace I've found by having no guilt and no striving. I've changed the colour of my hair and my two sons are very happy with what they see and hear from their new mum . . .

I'm so happy to find what I've always wanted. I didn't know that it was, or could be, possible – the reality of such a thing, to always live this way. But now I have found out, I'm always sharing whenever and however I can. It's much too good and wonderful to keep just for myself.'

Anyone who has now purchased one of my *Whole Body Programme* videos will be aware that exercising along with me is a delightful group of women who have very effectively slimmed down to present a picture of health and vitality and inspire all those who participate in the privacy of their own homes.

Joan Draycott was one of the girls who appeared in the first *Whole Body Programme* video. In 1991 I had the privilege of attending the wedding of Joan and Neil. The other girls in the video also attended and as Joan arrived in her magnificent wedding gown I could hardly speak. She looked so outstandingly beautiful, I wanted to take a picture of her and place it on the front cover of *Brides* magazine.

Joanne, her sister-in-law-to-be – Joan and Joanne are marrying two delightful guys who are brothers – was bridesmaid and she, too, looked gorgeous in her peach-coloured fitted dress. I was so proud of them. After the wedding Joan wrote to me. This is what she said:

'Just a short note to say a big thank-you for all your help with your wonderful diet. If it wasn't for you I would never have felt so nice on the happiest day of my life – my wedding day. I don't know if you can remember when you asked for a photo of me and few words saying why I wanted to lose weight. I wrote that the reason was because of my wedding day, but most of all I wished to be able to look back at the wedding photos showing I was 9½ st (60.3 kg), instead of 11½ st (73 kg). Well, I did it . . . and now I look at my photos and think, "Yes, I do look and feel great." I don't mean to be vain when I say that, but it is a wonderful feeling . . .'

Perhaps the most dramatic personality transformation was experienced by Helen, who wrote to me on 28 March. This is what she said:

'THANK YOU!!!

9 January – Went to sales, squeezing into size 16.
10 January – Your diet was in *Sunday Express*. Started immediately.

Up to this date, no social life, very conscious of overweight. I'm 5 ft 6 ins (1.68 m) but felt so

129

fat. Also, for long-ingrained reasons, terrified of being hungry.

19 March – Into size 12s. Confident enough to join Computer Dating Agency last week, all wanting to see me again.

24 March – Annual General Meeting at work. Surrounded by compliments. New hairstyle, make-up and glamorous specs.

I'm forty-nine this Thursday. The girls (average age twenty-three) have grabbed your book and it sits in the office. If this sounds like an advert, too bad. I'm happy and without being hungry!'

In my reply, I requested permission to reproduce Helen's letter – and also asked her if she would like to complete a questionnaire. She wrote back:

'Thank you for your kind letter. I have filled in the questionnaire in a way you might not find typical. When you read my replies you will see why.

You have full permission to publish my initial letter and perhaps the other history. Nobody is unique and it could be worth a chapter – even some dietitians/shrinks might be interested. Anonymity isn't important.

Last night, a nice man (younger than me!) expressed beautiful remarks about me physically and proposed. I may not accept, but this is down to your basic sense in making it possible.

Seems as though life may begin at forty-nine!

After a lifetime of eating disorders and totally abnormal attitudes to food, you have set me straight in two months. Mother would have apoplexy if she saw me now!'

When I read this letter, I could sense that Helen had gone through some very difficult times in her life. I could also see how successful she had been in following the diet. At 5 ft 6 ins (1.68 m) tall and wearing size 8 shoes it was clear that Helen was large-boned. In eleven weeks she had reduced her weight from 12 st 3 lbs to 9 st 6 lbs (77.7 to 60 kg). She had followed the diet extremely strictly, even cutting out bread and potatoes. This had not affected her health in any way and, she said, 'I feel wonderful and confident – run up stairs like a ten-year-old.'

Helen wanted to lose the heavy look on her face and she described the result: 'New face meant lovely new hairstyle – super make-up and new specs.'

She found the quick results and the encouragement she received from her work colleagues enabled her to enjoy following the diet. She hardly ever felt hungry and 'above all I can live sensibly with meals out as wanted'. She often used to binge, but never did whilst following the Hip and Thigh Diet.

In answer to the question: 'Were you more successful on this diet than with previous diets?' Helen ticked YES, with six ticks! 'I didn't feel hungry, of which I have a horror – see below,' she wrote. Then she told me about her tragic earlier life.

'*Age 10–16*: Mother starved me. She hated father, said he was all she could get because she was fat when young. At ten, I was attacked for "stealing" slice of bread. Public weighings at the chemist's with hysterical outbursts if up 4 ozs (100 g). Friends at school pitied me.

Age 16–31: Kept severely "controlled". Her sadism was matched by ignorance. Simultaneously

131

"protected" from young men, my being saved for her old age. Food was heaven when I got it.

Age 31: Left home, orgy of eating.

Age 40: Still all potential husbands manipulated off. Career brilliant. 15 st (95.4 kg), crash dieted on diet of Coke/black coffee.

Age 40 + 8 months: 8½ st (54 kg).

Age 40–48: Alternated anorexia and bulimia – down to under 7 st (44.5 kg). (By now unable to sustain hunger.) In and out of hospital. Career in limbo as tied to mother.

Age 48: Broke from mother. Bingeing, new happy job, content, undisciplined about eating – cheese, butter, etc. Feeling unattractive. Size 16+.

Age 48+: 10 January Sales, size 16+.
11 January Started diet.
(Eating now a nice normal feature, not a career!)
9 March: Shopped, size 12. Enrolled in marriage bureau.
24 March: 49th birthday.
26 March: First proposal – and now found sexually desirable.

I am happy. Flat being renovated like me! *Life is great!*'

7
Thighs of Relief – Hip, Hip, Hooray!

What the questionnaires told me

I can remember the sheer joy I felt when, after the first trial of the diet, the completed questionnaires began dropping through my letter-box. The air of enthusiasm and excitement from the trial team spurred me on tremendously as I wrote my first *Hip and Thigh Diet* book.

You can imagine my delight when again, after the book was published, people started writing to tell me how successful they had found the diet. I had never considered writing a follow-up *Complete Hip and Thigh Diet* book, but as time went by and more ideas for meals were requested it became clear that a follow-up book was inevitable, plus another cookery book, exercise cassette and a new video.

Questionnaires were issued to anyone who would be kind enough to complete one. Very conveniently we have a computer company located close to our office and they prepared a document which drew out comprehensive statistical information in a very readable and understandable format.

This chapter details the results of these completed questionnaires.

The initial analysis from which I commenced writing my second book was based on the results of 129 completed questionnaires. As my book approached completion I updated the statistics with the results from another sixty questionnaires which I had received in the meantime. It is fascinating to realize that the attitudes, opinions and results are virtually unchanged, though the number of responses has greatly increased. From the first book this was excellent news, because it indicated that despite the number of original volunteers who had kindly completed questionnaires being really quite small, the results were consistent and they were very interesting indeed.

The majority were completed by women in the middle age range, 35–64, falling in almost equal quantities into the 35–44, 45–54 and 55–64 age ranges. Twenty-five % described themselves as 'very overweight', 43% said they were 'quite overweight', 28% described themselves as 'slightly overweight' and 4.0% were 'not overweight' but wished to reduce inches.

The average time of following the diet was ten weeks and the average weight loss was 19 lbs (8.6 kg). Forty-seven % said they followed the diet 'very strictly', 51% said 'moderately strictly', and 2% said 'not very strictly'.

I asked the computer to segregate the 'strict' slimmers and to calculate their average weight loss. Not surprisingly it was proved that those who followed the diet 'very strictly' lost an average of 22 lbs (10 kg) over the average ten-week period, with those who followed it 'moderately strictly' losing 16 lbs (7.3 kg). Those who were following the diet 'not very strictly' still managed to lose 11 lbs (5 kg) over the average ten-week period.

Another aspect in which I was very interested was related to the fact that I had allowed a couple of alcoholic drinks per day to be consumed within the diet. We extracted from the computer those who said they had consumed their alcohol allowance *and* had followed the diet 'very strictly' and their average weight loss over ten weeks was 17 lbs (7.7 kg). We further investigated this question and discovered that the 'very strict' dieters who drank only occasionally lost the most – 24 lbs (10.9 kg) and those who were non-drinkers but stuck 'strictly' to the diet actually lost only a little less, losing an average of 23 lbs (10.4 kg).

From this it is easy to see that an occasional drink can actually be helpful to the dieter. I think this is because a drink in the evening can serve to relax us and we therefore feel less inclined to nibble. Bearing this in mind, and to encourage maximum possible weight loss combined with greatest possible freedom, I have modified the alcohol allowance to one per day for women, with three extra drinks per week to be taken when appropriate within one's social activities. Men may have two drinks per day plus three extra per week. See Chapter 8 for full details.

I have already, in Chapter 3, detailed the inch loss statistics and the areas of the body from which dieters lost the inches, so I will not repeat them, wonderful though the results were! Here are the answers to the other questions not mentioned elsewhere.

Do you think your cellulite has reduced? I asked.

A few didn't answer the question, but of the remainder, 57% said a definite 'Yes', 8% said 'No' and the remaining 31% said they didn't know.

Cellulite is the ghastly dimpled flesh usually found on women (and not necessarily overweight women) around thighs, hips and upper arms. It is ugly because it gives an uneven appearance to the skin, creating actual cavities in the flesh if pinched; an 'orange-peel' effect is another term used to describe it. I had experienced a dramatic improvement on my own legs when I first embarked on my diet for health reasons. I used to call myself 'Miss Cellulite 198—' according to the year! It was a constant source of real embarrassment. When I followed my very low-fat diet, I didn't eliminate the presence of cellulite, but it was significantly improved. I was glad to see that so many Hip and Thigh Dieters had experienced similar results. Jo Hodgart, for example, wrote: 'I had *terrible* "orange-peel" thighs, but they are almost normal now.'

Did you feel healthier as a result of following this diet?

I was interested to know how people had felt since following my diet. A resounding 89% stated they felt healthier, with only 1% saying they didn't feel better, 10% said there was 'no change' in the way they felt.

In answer to this question *What was the effect of the diet on hair, nails and skin?* these were the results:

	Improved	Deteriorated	Same
Hair	33.6%	2.8%	63.0%
Nails	29.2%	7.6%	63.2%
Skin	41.4%	2.0%	56.6%

I think if you had asked everyone before they embarked on the diet what the effects *might* be, the answers would almost certainly have been 'deterioration' on all counts because we were changing our eating habits so dramatically. I was delighted with such a positive result: a far greater degree of *improvement*, compared with very little deterioration. This would seem further to confirm that the Hip and Thigh Diet really is a healthy one. Often we can experience a deterioration in the condition of our hair and skin within *days* if we are unwell. So to see such a degree of improvement in such a short period of time must be encouraging and comforting to anyone who has doubts. Helena Livingstone wrote:

'One thing I must thank you for is the massive improvement in my skin. It always used to be very dingy and blotchy but now it glows! So much so that people have actually commented upon it!'

I asked my slimmers if they enjoyed following this diet. Everyone, except one gentleman, answered YES. (I rather think he had been forced on to it by his wife. Oh dear!)

In answer to the question about alcohol consumption, 30.8% said they did drink their alcohol allowance; 42.8% said they did 'occasionally', whilst 26% did not.

I asked if my volunteers had been following a diet before embarking on the Hip and Thigh Diet. 19.6% had been dieting recently but the remainder had not. 11.2% said it was their first attempt at dieting, 45.2% said they had dieted very occasionally in the past and 43.2% admitted trying more diets than they cared to remember! *An amazing 90.8% said they were more successful on this diet*; 1.2% said they were not more successful. Some, of course, abstained from answering the question because they had never dieted before.

So why was the Hip and Thigh Diet more successful? As we discussed in an earlier chapter, dieters said it was mainly because it was easy to follow; they could eat so much more than on most diets; because it didn't involve any calorie counting; and because they could *see* the results so quickly. A great number of the questionnaires I received included the spontaneous comment from slimmers that 'this didn't seem like a diet; it is more a way of eating'. I think that really sums up why it is so incredibly successful – diets fail because the slimmer feels over-disciplined, deprived and hungry. With the Hip and Thigh Diet you don't experience any of these feelings.

This was further proved by a separate trial which was organized by *The Journal* newspaper in Newcastle upon Tyne. During my initial book promotional tour I had a very enjoyable interview with a charming lady called Avril Deane who at that time was the Women's Page Editor. When she suggested her own trial, run through the newspaper, I couldn't help feeling that Avril was waiting for me to hesitate and question whether this was a good idea. Naturally, knowing how effective the diet was, I was all for putting it to the test yet again. *Journal* readers were asked to write in and twelve were selected to follow the diet, for eight weeks. I had no contact with them whatsoever.

In early June the following piece appeared in *The Journal*.

THIGHS OF RELIEF AND HIP HIP HOORAY!

Words of praise from readers for writer Rosemary Conley and her Hip and Thigh Diet which we featured in February . . .

The no-fat diet, specially for pear-shaped people, has helped them shed stones (many kilos) of unwanted weight and now they are persuading their friends to give it a go.

'I've lost a stone (6.4 kg) in eight weeks and I'm really pleased,' says Mrs Maureen Rumfitt, who was one of our dozen volunteers who agreed to try out the diet.

'I'm going on holiday soon and I'm keeping on with it until I reach the right weight. I've tried other diets and usually the weight has come straight off my bust.

Maureen, 42, and a mother of four grown-up children, had despaired of losing weight on her thighs and hips.

For Mrs Sandra Kitching, 26, with a year-old daughter, the diet has helped her get down to her ideal size by getting rid of a surplus stone (6.4 kg).

'I lost the weight in six weeks and most of the time it was quite easy to stick to the diet. Occasionally I fancied a bit of chocolate but there was plenty to eat and I certainly wasn't starving,' says Sandra who lives in Jarrow.

Capheaton postmistress Mrs Sheila Davidson managed to lose one stone and six pounds (9.1 kg) during the first eight weeks and is persevering to lose another stone (6.4 kg) at least.

Her downfall was nibbling sweets while she was working in the post office and she was delighted with the way she lost her desire for margarine and butter and other fats.

But she confesses: 'Although I haven't had many sweets I still miss slices of cake at the weekends especially when the kids are eating them.'

Detailed questionnaires filled in by our readers who have been trying out the diet are being sent to Rosemary Conley who has promised she will try and include them in her next book. Many thanks to you all!

At the time of writing the first edition of *Complete Hip and Thigh Diet* book, I had actually received only two questionnaires (apparently the trial team had been interviewed on the telephone for the article). The two volunteers who did write to me in time to be included were Alison Hall and Linda Towns. Alison wrote:

'I measured myself prior to diet, and sent details to Avril Deane. I felt if I had to measure myself, that would put me off going any further. I tried on all the clothes that I haven't been able to wear for at least two years, and found *that* a better incentive to carry on. This diet means I can concentrate on living my life, without the worry of "what can I have and what I can't" to eat. I can thoroughly recommend this diet to anyone overweight. This diet has certainly taught me a healthy way to eat, without the need for pills, etc., in order to lose weight.'

Alison lost 11 lbs (5 kg). She lost 2 ins (5 cm) from her bust, 3½ ins (9 cm) from her waist, 3 ins (8 cm) from her hips, 3 ins (7.5 cm) from one thigh and 2 ins (5 cm) from the other.

Linda Towns reduced her weight from 10 st 5 lbs to 8 st 9 lbs (66 to 55 kg) and said:

'I haven't been this weight for at least thirteen years. I'm going on holiday soon and I hope I can be good. I shall return to the diet after my holiday knowing at last I've found a diet that really works with not *too* great an effort.'

Along with her 24 lbs (10.9 kg) weight loss, Linda lost 2 ins (5 cm) from her bust, 4 ins (10 cm) from her waist, 4 ins (10 cm) from her hips and almost 3 ins (8 cm) from each thigh, 2 ins (5 cm) from her knees and over 1 inch (2.5 cm) from each arm. No wonder she was pleased!

8

The Diet – extended version

The diet described in the following pages is based on the original diet followed by my initial trial team, amended to cater for the discerning tastes of those who followed it, and now extended to incorporate all possible social demands whether they be on economic grounds or the practical need of taking a packed lunch to work. In this book I have also catered for vegetarians.

This diet includes many new menu suggestions, but for your convenience I have also repeated all the menu suggestions from the first Hip and Thigh Diet. The result is a vast variety of food to satisfy every possible taste, for those with a large appetite, those with a tiny one, those who like cooking and those who like to keep it simple. As you become more familiar with the fat content of foods by studying the very comprehensive fat tables in Chapter 14 you will soon be able to formulate your own diet menus. I have included a list of strictly forbidden foods within this chapter to enable you to make a definite resolution (*before* you commence the diet) to ban them. If you are going to cheat and sneak bars of chocolate or packets of salted peanuts into your cupboard to eat when nobody's looking, you might as well give this book to somebody else. It has been *proved* that this diet will help you achieve the kind of figure-shape you never dreamed possible, but there is only one person in the world who can actually make it work for you – and that's YOU.

Perhaps the best news for slimmers is that this diet gives you a greater volume of food than any other reducing diet, and gives you lots of freedom. You are allowed three meals a day and an alcoholic drink too into the bargain! You will be staggered how quickly you see results, both in weight and inch loss, and this will encourage you to continue. The additional energy and generally healthier feeling that was enjoyed by so many of those who wrote to me, or completed questionnaires, showed they had a real sense of happiness and contentment. It was wonderful for me to read about it and no doubt tremendous for those who experienced such success.

Just think – this is almost certainly going to be the last time you ever have to diet! Can you imagine how wonderful that will be? So go for it! You've got nothing to lose but those inches.

Diet instructions

Eat three meals a day, selecting one meal from the Breakfast, Lunch and Dinner menus listed. The dinner menus offer three courses. These may be broken up to provide a snack for later in the day if necessary, but try if possible to stick to the three-meals-a-day routine.

Daily allowance
10 fl oz (½ pint) [250 ml] skimmed or semi-skimmed milk

1 alcoholic drink for women, 2 for men, plus 3 extra per week (optional)
4 fl oz (100 ml) unsweetened fruit juice

Diet notes
'Unlimited vegetables' includes potatoes as well as all other vegetables provided they are cooked and served without fat. Pasta, provided it is egg-free and fat-free, may be substituted for potatoes, rice or similar carbohydrate food.

'One piece of fruit' means one average apple or one orange, etc., or approximately 4 oz (100 g) in weight, e.g. a 4 oz (100 g) slice of pineapple.

Red meat: Don't forget to restrict red meat to just two helpings a week.

Gravy may be taken with dinner menus provided it is made with gravy powder, not granules. Do not add meat juices from the roasting tin unless you first discard the fat (see recipe, page 284).

All yogurts should be the low-calorie, low-fat, diet brands. Cottage cheese should be the low-fat variety.

Jacket potatoes are stated without a weight restriction. Use your own discretion in order to satisfy your appetite (see my comments in Chapter 2).

'Light' bread means brands such as Slimcea or Nimble.

Between-meal snacks
Chopped cucumber, celery, carrots, tomatoes and peppers may be consumed between meals if necessary.

The diet

Part 1	Breakfasts:	*Cereal breakfasts*
		Fruit breakfasts
		Cooked and continental breakfasts
Part 2	Lunches:	*Fruit lunches*
		Packed lunches
		Cold lunches
		Hot lunches
Part 3	Dinners:	*Starters*
		Main courses: non-vegetarian
		Main courses: vegetarian
		Additional notes for vegetarians
		Desserts
		Drinks
		Sauces and dressings
Part 4	Daily nutritional requirements	
Part 5	The forbidden list	
Part 6	The binge corrector menu	

Part 1: Breakfasts

Select any one

Cereal breakfasts

v = *Suitable for vegetarians*

The following may be served with skimmed milk from allowance and 1 teaspoon brown sugar if desired.

1. **v** 1 oz (25 g) porridge oats, made with water, served with 2 teaspoons honey, no sugar.
2. **v** Home-made muesli (see recipe, page 178).
3. **v** 1 oz (25 g) Branflakes or Fruit 'n' Fibre.
4. **v** 1 oz (25 g) Cornflakes, Puffed Rice, Sugarflakes or Rye and Raisin Cereal.
5. **v** 2 Weetabix.
6. **v** 1 oz (25 g) wholewheat cereal.
7. **v** ¾ oz (18.75 g) All Bran, plus ½ oz (12.5 g) Fruit 'n' Fibre.
8. **v** ¾ oz (18.75 g) All Bran, plus 1 small banana, sliced.
9. **v** Any one Variety Pack, plus 2 oz (50 g) chopped fresh fruit.
10. **v** ½ oz (12.5 g) Branflakes, ½ oz (12.5 g) sultanas mixed with a 5 oz (125 g) diet yogurt.
11. **v** ½ oz (12.5 g) branded muesli, plus ½ oz (12.5 g) All Bran, no sugar.

Fruit breakfasts

v = *Suitable for vegetarians*

NB 'Diet yogurt' means low-fat, low-calorie yogurt.

1. **v** 1 banana plus 5 oz (125 g) diet yogurt – any flavour.
2. **v** 4 oz (100 g) tinned peaches in natural juice plus 5 oz (125 g) diet yogurt – any flavour.
3. **v** 5 tinned prunes in natural juice plus 5 oz (125 g) natural yogurt.
4. **v** 5 tinned prunes in natural juice, plus half a slice of toast, plus 1 teaspoon marmalade.
5. **v** 4 dried apricots, soaked (see recipe for Stewed Apricots or Prunes, page 178), plus 5 oz (125 g) diet yogurt – any flavour.
6. **v** As much fresh fruit as you can eat at one sitting.
7. **v** 5 oz (125 g) stewed fruit (cooked without sugar), plus diet yogurt – any flavour.
8. **v** 6 oz (150 g) fruit compote (e.g. oranges, grapefruit, peaches, pineapple, pears – all in natural juice).
9. **v** 8 oz (200 g) tinned grapefruit in natural juice.
10. **v** 1 whole fresh grapefruit, plus 5 oz (125 g) diet yogurt – any flavour.
11. **v** Half a melon topped with a 5 oz (125 g) diet yogurt.
12. **v** 1 wedge of melon topped with 3 oz (75 g) grapes and served with 2 oz (50 g) diet yogurt.

cont.

Fruit breakfasts cont.

13. **v** 4 oz (100 g) strawberries, plus 4 oz (100 g) melon, chopped, and topped with 2 oz (50 g) diet yogurt.
14. **v** 8 oz (200 g) raspberries or strawberries topped with 5 oz (125 g) diet yogurt.
15. **v** 6 oz (150 g) fresh fruit salad topped with 5 oz (125 g) diet yogurt.
16. **v** 1 large slice fresh pineapple, plus 4 oz (100 g) strawberries topped with 2 oz (50 g) diet yogurt.
17. **v** Chop 1 banana and stir into 5 oz (125 g) diet yogurt – any flavour. Add ½ oz (12.5 g) All Bran cereal and mix well.
18. **v** Banana Milk Shake (see recipe, page 178).
19. **v** Banana and Orange Cocktail (see recipe 179).
20. **v** 1 slice of Banana and Sultana Cake (see recipe, page 276).
21. **v** 3 green figs, plus 3 oz (75 g) diet yogurt.

Cooked and continental breakfasts

v = *Suitable for vegetarians*

1. **v** 8 oz (200 g) baked beans served on 1 slice (1 oz/25 g) toast.
2. **v** 8 oz (200 g) tinned tomatoes served on 1 slice (1½ oz/37.5 g) toast.
3. 2 oz (50 g) very lean bacon (all fat removed) served with unlimited tinned tomatoes.
4. **v** Half a grapefruit, plus 1 slice (1½ oz/37.5 g) toast with 2 teaspoons marmalade.
5. 8 oz (200 g) smoked haddock, steamed in skimmed milk.
6. 2 oz (50 g) lean ham, 2 tomatoes, plus 1 fresh wholemeal roll.
7. 2 oz (50 g) cured chicken or turkey breast or smoked turkey, 2 tomatoes, plus 1 fresh wholemeal roll.
8. 1 oz (25 g) very lean bacon (all fat removed) served with 4 oz (100 g) mushrooms cooked in vegetable stock, 3 oz (75 g) baked beans, 8 oz (200 g) tinned tomatoes or 4 fresh tomatoes grilled.
9. 1 oz (25 g) very lean bacon (all fat removed), 4 oz (100 g) mushrooms cooked in stock, 8 oz (200 g) tinned tomatoes or 4 fresh tomatoes grilled, plus half a slice (¾ oz/18.75 g) toast.
10. **v** 1 oz (25 g) wholemeal toast spread with Marmite and topped with 2 oz (50 g) cottage cheese.
11. **v** 4 Ryvitas spread with 1 tablespoon marmalade or preserve.

cont.

Cooked and continental breakfasts cont.

12. **v** Half a grapefruit, plus 3 Ryvitas spread with Marmite and topped with 2 oz (50 g) cottage cheese.

13. 1 slice light bread toasted, topped with 4 oz (100 g) baked beans mixed with 1 oz (25 g) lean ham, chopped, plus 1 tomato.

14. **v** 1 slice wholemeal toast spread with 1 teaspoon raspberry jam and topped with fine slices of one small banana. To add a luxury taste spoon 2 teaspoons low-fat fromage frais over banana slices if desired.

Part 2: Lunches

Select any one

Fruit lunches

v = *Suitable for vegetarians*

1. **v** Pineapple Boat (see recipe, page 179).
2. **v** Prawn and Grapefruit Cocktail (see recipe, page 180).
3. **v** 4–5 pieces any fruit (e.g. 1 orange, 1 apple, 1 pear, 4 oz [100 g] plums).
4. **v** 8 oz (200 g) fresh fruit salad topped with 5 oz (125 g) low-fat yogurt.
5. **v** 2 pieces any fresh fruit plus 2 × 5 oz (2 × 125 g) diet yogurts.
6. **v** 2 pears peeled, cored and brushed in lemon juice. Fill core cavities with 4 oz (100 g) cottage cheese and serve on a bed of lettuce.
7. **v** Cheese and Strawberry Pears (see recipe, page 181).
8. **v** 1 large Baked Stuffed Apple (see recipe, page 279), plus 5 oz (125 g) diet yogurt.
9. **v** Slice and serve together 2 medium bananas and 2 kiwifruits and top with 3 oz (75 g) low-fat fromage frais – any flavour.
10. **v** Fruit Sundae (see recipe, page 266).
11. Fruit and Chicken Salad (see recipe, page 183).
12. Kiwifruit and Ham Salad (see recipe, page 185).
13. **v** Orange and Carrot Salad (see recipe, pages 185–6).

cont.

Fruit lunches cont.

14. **v** Summer Delight (see recipe, pages 181–2).
15. **v** 1 lb (400 g) strawberries or raspberries, plus diet yogurt.
16. **v** Stilton Pears (see recipe, pages 180–1).

Packed lunches

v = Suitable for vegetarians

1. 2 slices bread, spread with reduced-oil salad dressing, piled with lettuce, salad and prawns.
2. **v** Contents of small tin baked beans, plus chopped salad of lettuce, tomatoes, onions, celery, cucumber.
3. 2 slices bread with 1 oz (25 g) ham, 1 tomato and pickle.
4. 4 Ryvitas spread with 2 oz (50 g) pickle and 4 slices of turkey roll or chicken roll, or 3 oz (75 g) ordinary chicken or turkey breast, plus 2 tomatoes. 1 piece of fruit.
5. Chicken leg (no skin), chopped salad (lettuce, tomatoes, onions, celery, cucumber), soy sauce or Worcestershire sauce plus natural yogurt.
6. 4 Ryvitas, low-fat cottage cheese, topped with prawns.
7. **v** 4 Ryvitas, spread thinly with low-fat soft cheese and topped with salad.
8. **v** 4 oz (100 g) red kidney beans, 4 oz (100 g) sweetcorn, plus chopped cucumber, tomatoes, onions tossed in mint sauce and natural yogurt.
9. **v** 4 × 5 oz (4 × 125 g) low-fat, low-calorie yogurts – any flavour.

cont.

Packed lunches cont.

10. Salad of lettuce, tomato, cucumber, onion, grated carrot, etc., plus prawns, shrimps, lobster or crab (6 oz/150 g total seafood) and Seafood Dressing (see recipes 1 and 2, pages 281–2).

11. **v** 4 Ryvitas, spread with any flavour low-fat cottage cheese, topped with tomatoes plus unlimited salad vegetables.

12. 1 slimmers' cup-a-soup. 2 Ryvitas spread with low-fat cottage cheese or soft cheese topped with salad vegetables. 5 oz (125 g) diet yogurt.

13. 1 slimmers' cup-a-soup. 2 pieces fresh fruit. 5 oz (125 g) diet yogurt.

14. 1 slimmers' cup-a-soup. 2 slices light bread, spread with 2 teaspoons reduced-oil salad dressing and topped with salad and 2 oz (50 g) cottage cheese.

15. Triple-decker sandwich – composed of 3 slices light bread filled with 1 oz (25 g) turkey or chicken breast roll, or 2 oz (50 g) cottage cheese, lettuce, tomatoes, cucumber, sliced Spanish onion. Spread bread with oil-free sweet pickle of your choice, e.g. Branston or similar, or mustard, ketchup or reduced-oil salad dressing.

16. 3 Ryvitas spread with 2 oz (50 g) pilchards in tomato sauce, topped with sliced tomato.

17. 2 slices wholemeal bread spread with Seafood Dressing (see recipes 1 & 2, pages 281–2) and made into sandwiches with 2 oz (50 g) tinned salmon and cucumber.

18. 1 Pot Rice, plus 5 oz (150 g) diet yogurt.

Packed lunches cont.

19. **v** 4 slices light bread made into jumbo sandwiches. Spread bread with reduced-oil salad dressing and fill with lots of salad vegetables, e.g. lettuce, cucumber, onion, cress, tomatoes, beetroot, green and red peppers.
20. **v** Rice salad: a bowl of chopped peppers, tomatoes, onion, peas, sweetcorn and cucumber mixed with cooked (boiled) brown rice and served with soy sauce.
21. **v** 3 slices light bread or 4 Ryvitas spread with Marmite and 3 oz (75 g) cottage cheese.
22. **v** 1 bread roll, plus 2 oz (50 g) cottage cheese – any flavour – and unlimited vegetables.
23. 1 pack prepared salad (Marks & Spencer, Tesco, etc.), plus 4 oz (100 g) lean ham or 4 oz (100 g) skinless chicken or 6 oz (150 g) cottage cheese.
24. 4 Ryvitas spread with 3 oz (75 g) salmon, tuna or mackerel mixed with 1 tablespoon reduced-oil salad dressing, plus lettuce, tomato and cucumber.
25. 1 wholemeal roll (2 oz/50 g) spread only with mustard or pickle and filled with 1 oz (25 g) ham or chicken and salad.
26. **v** 1 slice Kim's Cake (see recipe, pages 275–6) or Banana and Sultana Cake (see recipe), page 276), plus 1 piece fresh fruit and 5 oz (125 g) diet yogurt.
27. Tuna Loaf with salad (see recipe, page 191).

Cold lunches

v = Suitable for vegetarians

1. Curried Chicken and Yogurt Salad (see recipe, page 182).
2. Seafood Salad (see recipe, page 184).
3. Cheese, Prawn and Asparagus Salad (see recipe, pages 184–5).
4. Chicken joint (with skin removed) or prawns, served with a chopped salad of lettuce, cucumber, radish, spring onions, mushrooms, peppers, tomatoes, with soy sauce or Yogurt Dressing (see recipe, page 281).
5. Crab and asparagus open sandwiches: 2 slices wholemeal bread spread with Seafood Dressing (see recipes 1 & 2, pages 281–2). Spread fresh or tinned crab meat or seafood sticks on to the bread and decorate with asparagus spears.
6. **v** Red Kidney Bean Salad (see recipe, page 187).
7. **v** 4 oz (100 g) cottage cheese (any flavour), served with large assorted salad and Carrot Salad (see recipe, page 185).
8. Large salad served with prawns, plus Carrot Salad (see recipe, page 185) dressed with low-fat natural yogurt.
9. **v** 8 oz (200 g) carton low-fat cottage cheese, with two tinned pear halves, chopped apple and celery, served on a bed of lettuce and garnished with tomato and cucumber.

Cold lunches cont.

10. 3 oz (75 g) pilchards served in tomato sauce, or tuna in brine or salmon, served with a large salad and Oil-free Orange and Lemon Vinaigrette dressing (see recipe, page 280).
11. 3 oz (75 g) salmon served with a large salad and mint yogurt dressing.
12. Mixed salad served with 4 oz (100 g) diet coleslaw – any flavour plus 4 oz (100 g) low-calorie potato salad, plus 2 oz (50 g) prawns or 2 oz (50 g) chicken.
13. **v** 4 Ryvitas spread with low-calorie coleslaw – any flavour – and topped with salad.
14. **v** 15 oz (375 g) tin baked beans, served cold, with salad. No dressing.
15. **v** Bean Salad (see recipe, page 186).
16. **v** Mash one banana with 2 oz (50 g) cottage cheese and spread it on a thin slice of wholemeal bread. Top with another slice of bread, cut into triangles and serve immediately.
17. **v** Chilli Salad (see recipe, page 188).
18. **v** Chinese Apple Salad (see recipe, pages 187–8).
19. 2 oz (50 g) ham or chicken with 8 oz (200 g) Coleslaw (see recipe, pages 262–3).
20. Curried Chicken and Yogurt Salad (see recipe, page 182).
21. Tomato Galantine (see recipe, pages 188–9).

Hot lunches

v = Suitable for vegetarians

1. **v** Jacket potato topped with 8 oz (200 g) tin baked beans.
2. **v** 2 slices light bread toast topped with 15 oz (375 g) tin baked beans.
3. **v** Jacket potato served with 3 oz (75 g) low-fat cottage cheese and salad (cottage cheese may be flavoured with chives, onion, pineapple, etc., but it must be 'low fat').
4. **v** Clear or vegetable soup, served with 1 oz (25 g) slice toast followed by 2 pieces of fruit.
5. Jacket potato with 1 oz (25 g) roast beef, pork or ham (with all fat removed) or 2 oz (50 g) chicken (no skin), served with Branston pickle and salad.
6. **v** 2 slices wholemeal toast with small tin baked beans and small tin tomatoes.
7. **v** Jacket potato served with sweetcorn and chopped salad.
8. **v** Jacket potato served with grated carrot, chopped onion, tomatoes, sweetcorn and peppers, topped with natural yogurt.
9. **v** Jacket potato filled with 4 oz (100 g) cottage cheese mixed with 4 teaspoons tomato purée and black pepper to taste.
10. Jacket potato with Barbecue Topping (see recipe, pages 194–5).
11. Jacket potato with Chilli Bacon (see recipe, page 196).
12. Club Sandwich (see recipe, pages 189–90).

Hot lunches cont.

13. **v** Mixed Vegetable Soup (see recipe, pages 192–3), plus 2 oz (50 g) wholemeal roll.
14. **v** Boil 8 oz (200 g) tinned tomatoes and 3 oz (75 g) tinned button mushrooms together, vigorously, in a non-stick pan until they reach a creamy consistency. Place on top of 2 slices hot wholemeal toast. Season with freshly ground black pepper.
15. **v** Potato Madras (see recipe, page 196).
16. Jacket Potato with Chicken and Peppers (see recipe, page 195).
17. Jacket Potato with Chopped Vegetables (see recipe, page 194).
18. Jacket Potato with Prawns and Sweetcorn (see recipe, page 195).
19. **v** 2 oz (50 g) Tofu Burger (see recipe, page 261), served with large salad.
20. **v** Stuffed Marrow (see recipe, page 254).
21. **v** Stuffed Pepper (see recipe, page 197).
22. Chicken Liver Salad (see recipe, pages 182–3).
23. **v** Oat and Cheese Loaf (see recipe, page 260).
24. **v** Oriental Stir-fry (see recipe, pages 197–8).
25. **v** 2 oz (50 g) wholemeal toast topped with 8 oz (200 g) can spaghetti in tomato sauce.
26. Fish Chowder (see recipe, pages 193–4).
27. Fresh Vegetable Soup (see recipe, page 192) plus 1 slice toast.

Part 3: Dinners

Select any one from each category:
Starters
Main courses
(vegetarian or non-vegetarian)
Side dishes
Desserts

Starters

v = *Suitable for vegetarians*

1. **v** Crudités (see recipe, page 198).
2. Chicken and Mushroom Soup (see recipe, page 208).
3. **v** Orange and Grapefruit Cocktail (see recipe, page 199).
4. Melon and Prawn Salad (see recipe, page 200).
5. **v** Pair of Pears (see recipe, page 200).
6. **v** French Tomatoes (see recipe, pages 200–1).
7. **v** Grapefruit segments in natural juice.
8. **v** Melon balls in slimline ginger ale.
9. Clear soup.
10. **v** Garlic Mushrooms (see recipe, pages 202–3).
11. **v** Melon Salad (see recipe, pages 201–2).
12. **v** Ratatouille (see recipe, page 203).
13. **v** Wedge of melon.
14. **v** Half a grapefruit.
15. **v** Grilled Grapefruit (see recipe, page 199).
16. Beef and Vegetable Soup (see recipe, pages 207–8).
17. Chicken Soup (see recipe, pages 208–9).

Starters cont.

18. Duck Soup (see recipe, pages 209–10).
19. **v** Creamy Vegetable Soup (see recipe, page 204).
20. **v** Butter Bean and Carrot Soup (see recipe, page 205).
21. **v** Leek and Potato Soup (see recipe, pages 204–5).
22. **v** Creamy Mushroom Soup (see recipe, pages 205–6).
23. **v** Curried Courgette Soup (see recipe, pages 206–7).
24. **v** Curried Potato and Parsnip Soup (see recipe, page 206).

Main courses: non-vegetarian

1. Stir-fried Chicken and Vegetables (see recipe, pages 222–3).
2. Snapper Florentine (see recipe, pages 233–4) with unlimited vegetables.
3. Chicken Veronique (see recipe, pages 229–30) with Lyonnaise Potatoes (see recipe, page 247) and unlimited vegetables.
4. Tandoori Chicken (see recipe, page 226).
5. Shepherd's Pie (see recipe, pages 210–11).
6. Fish Curry with rice (see recipe, page 235).
7. Steak Surprise (see recipe, page 219) plus jacket potato, boiled mushrooms, and unlimited vegetables.
8. 8 oz (200 g) steamed, grilled or microwaved white fish (cod, plaice, whiting, haddock, lemon sole, halibut) served with unlimited boiled vegetables.
9. 8 oz (200 g) chicken joint (weighed cooked including the bones), baked with skin removed, in Barbecue Sauce (see recipe, page 282) and served with jacket potato or boiled brown rice and vegetables of your choice.
10. Chicken Chinese-style (see recipe, page 224).
11. Spaghetti Bolognese (see recipes 1 & 2, pages 211–13).
12. Barbecued Chicken or Turkey Kebabs (see recipe, pages 227–8) served with boiled brown rice.
13. 3 oz (75 g) roast leg of pork with all fat removed, served with apple sauce and unlimited vegetables.

Main courses: non-vegetarian cont.

14. Steamed or grilled or microwaved trout, stuffed with prawns and served with a large salad or assorted vegetables.
15. 6 oz (150 g) calves' or lamb's liver, braised with onions, and served with unlimited vegetables.
16. 6 oz (150 g) turkey (no skin) served with cranberry sauce, Dry-roast Potatoes (see recipe, page 264), and unlimited vegetables.
17. 3 oz (75 g) roast lamb with all fat removed, served with Dry-roast Parsnips (see recipe, page 264) and unlimited vegetables.
18. 6 oz (150 g) chicken (no skin) steamed, grilled, baked or microwaved, and served with unlimited vegetables.
19. Chicken or Prawn Chop Suey (see recipe, pages 223–4) served with boiled brown rice.
20. Chicken Curry (see recipe, pages 226–7) served with boiled brown rice.
21. 3 oz (75 g) grilled or baked gammon steak or gammon rashers, with all fat removed, served with pineapple and unlimited vegetables.
22. Fish Pie (see recipe, pages 234–5) served with unlimited vegetables.
23. Chicken Fricassée (see recipe, page 229).
24. 4 oz (100 g) roast duck (all skin removed) served with unlimited vegetables.
25. Chinese Chicken (see recipe, page 224).
26. Fish Risotto (see recipe, pages 235–6).
27. Coq au Vin (see recipe, pages 232–3).

cont.

Main courses: non-vegetarian cont.

28. Dijon-style Kidneys (see recipe, pages 220–1).
29. Fillet Steaks with Green Peppercorns (see recipe, pages 219–20).
30. Mussels in White Wine (see recipe, page 236).
31. Spicy Meatballs (see recipe, pages 215–16).
32. Steak and Kidney Pie (see recipe, pages 218–19).
33. Spaghetti Chicken (see recipe, pages 228–9).
34. Pork and Pear Sauce (see recipe, pages 221–2).
35. Mince and Spaghetti Casserole (see recipe, page 214).
36. Spicy Meat Loaf (see recipe, page 217).
37. Chilli con Carne (see recipe, page 215).
38. Lasagne (see recipe, pages 213–14).
39. Chicken à l'Orange (see recipe, pages 231–2).

Main courses: vegetarian

1. Chickpea Couscous (see recipe, pages 251–2).
2. Vegetable Bake (see recipe, page 238).
3. Vegetarian Shepherd's Pie (see recipe, page 165) served with unlimited vegetables.
4. Vegetable Curry (see recipe, page 241) served on a bed of boiled brown rice.
5. Vegetarian Chilli con Carne (see recipe, page 165) served on a bed of boiled brown rice.
6. Vegetable Chilli (see recipe, pages 242–3) served on a bed of boiled brown rice.
7. Vegetarian Spaghetti Bolognese (see recipe, pages 245–6).
8. Tricolour Pasta (see recipe, page 246).
9. Bean Salad (see recipe, page 186) served with cold boiled brown rice and soy sauce.
10. Hummus with Crudités (see recipe, pages 247–8).
11. Spiced Bean Casserole (see recipe, page 249) served with unlimited vegetables.
12. Vegetable Kebabs (see recipe, page 240) served on a bed of rice and sweetcorn.
13. Vegetable Casserole (see recipe, pages 238–9) served with boiled brown rice or Lyonnaise Potatoes (see recipe, page 247).
14. Three Bean Salad (see recipe, pages 248–9) served with salad and cold boiled brown rice.
15. Stuffed Peppers (see recipe, page 197) served with salad.

cont.

Main courses: vegetarian cont.

16. Blackeyed Bean Casserole (see recipe, pages 249–50).
17. Chickpea and Fennel Casserole (see recipe, pages 250–1).
18. Vegetable Chop Suey (see recipe, page 239) served with boiled brown rice.
19. Vegetarian Goulash (see recipe, pages 243–4).
20. Quarterpounder (100 g) Diet Burger, served with unlimited vegetables or large wholemeal bap.
21. Broccoli Delight (see recipe, pages 255–6).
22. Stir-fried Vegetables with Ginger and Sesame Marinade (see recipe, pages 257–8).
23. Hearty Hotpot (see recipe, pages 259–60).
24. Tofu Burgers (see recipe, page 261).
25. Oat and Cheese Loaf (see recipe, page 260).
26. Quick and Low-fat Courgette Lasagne (see recipe, pages 256–7).
27. Three-layer Millet Bake (see recipe, pages 252–3).
28. Mixed Grain and Fresh Coriander Medley (see recipe, pages 253–4).
29. Tofu Indonesian Style (see recipe, pages 261–2).
30. Fresh Tagliatelle with Blue Cheese Sauce (see recipe, pages 258–9).
31. Vegetable and Fruit Curry (see recipe, pages 241–2).

Additional notes for vegetarians

Vegetarians may include the following foods within menus designed by themselves or amended from the non-vegetarian dishes listed.

1 egg – 3 times a week.
1 oz (25 g) low-fat Edam cheese on non-egg days.
1 teaspoon oil may be used for cooking.
A few nuts and seeds – occasionally.

(The latter two are allowed 'in place of' fat in animal proteins such as meat, fish and poultry.)

A vegetarian diet is based on 5 major food groups, each of which should be regularly incorporated into your daily diet. These are: grains; pulses; nuts and seeds; dairy products; fruit and vegetables.

Grains
Barley
Buckwheat
Millet
Oats
Rice
Rye
Wheat
Wheat products such as flour, pasta, couscous, bulgar wheat

cont.

Additional notes for vegetarians cont.

Pulses
Aduki beans
Blackeyed beans
Brown lentils
Chickpeas
Mung beans
Peas
Red kidney beans
Red split lentils
Split peas

Nuts and seeds
These should be kept to a minimum, but a tiny amount is acceptable within this diet, for vegetarians only

Dairy products
These should be low-fat alternatives and include:
Low-fat cheese
Skimmed or semi-skimmed milk
Yogurt
Fromage frais

Fruits and vegetables
May be eaten freely at meal times

Desserts

1 teaspoon of diet yogurt or low-fat fromage frais
may be added to any of the following:

1. Meringue basket filled with raspberries and
   topped with raspberry yogurt or low-fat
   fromage frais.
2. Fruit Sundae (see recipe, page 266).
3. Baked Stuffed Apple (see recipe, page 279)
   served with plain yogurt.
4. 4 oz (100 g) fresh fruit salad mixed with 4 oz
   (100 g) diet yogurt.
5. Stewed fruit (cooked without sugar) served
   with 3 oz (75 g) Low-fat Custard (see
   recipe, pages 284–5).
6. Apple and Blackcurrant Whip (see recipe,
   page 269).
7. Pineapple and Orange Sorbet (see recipe,
   page 268).
8. Raspberry Mousse (see recipe, page 270).
9. Sliced banana topped with raspberry yogurt
   or low-fat fromage frais.
10. Fresh strawberries or raspberries served with
    diet yogurt.
11. Pears in Red Wine (see recipe, pages 270–1).
12. Pineapple in Kirsch (see recipe, page 272).
13. Oranges in Grand Marnier and Yogurt
    Sauce (see recipe, pages 272–3).
14. Sliced banana topped with fresh raspberries
    or strawberries.
15. Fresh peaches sliced and served with fresh
    raspberries.
16. Two pieces of fruit of your choice.

cont.

Desserts cont.

17. Pineapple Boat (see recipe, pages 179–80).
18. Diet Rice Pudding (see recipe, pages 278–9).
19. Fruit Sorbet (see recipe, page 267).
20. Pears in Meringue (see recipe, pages 271–2).
21. 8 oz (200 g) fresh fruit salad.
22. Peach Brûlée (see recipe, pages 274–5).
23. Stewed rhubarb sweetened with artificial sweetener, served with rhubarb diet yogurt.
24. Melon Sundae (see recipe, pages 266–7).
25. Hot Cherries and ice cream (see recipe, page 275).
26. Gooseberry Surprise (see recipe, pages 273–4).
27. 1 slice of Banana and Sultana Cake (see recipe, page 276).
28. 1 slice of Sultana Cake (see recipe, page 277).
29. Apple Jelly with Fromage Frais (see recipe, pages 268–9).
30. Fruit Jelly with Fromage Frais (see recipe, page 268).

Drinks

1. Orange/Lemon Barley Drink (see recipe, page 285). This is ideal for anyone allergic to artificial colourings or additives.
2. Pacific Delight (see recipe, page 286).
3. Apple Cola (see recipe, page 287).
4. Pineapple Sludge (see recipe, page 287).
5. Grapefruit Fizz (see recipe, page 286).
6. St Clements (see recipe, page 285).
7. Spritzer (see recipe, page 287).
8. Caribbean Surprise (see recipe, page 286).
9. Ginger Orange (see recipe, page 286).
10. Sludge Gulper (see recipe, page 287).
11. Buck's Fizz (see recipe, page 288).

Tea and coffee may be drunk freely if drunk black, or may be drunk white so long as milk allowance is not exceeded. Use artificial sweetener whenever possible in place of sugar.

Ladies may drink one alcoholic drink per day. Men may have two. One drink means a single measure of spirit, a glass of wine, or small glass of sherry or half a pint (250 ml) of beer or lager. 'Diet' drinks may be drunk freely.

You may drink as much water as you like; sparkling mineral water tastes wonderful.

Grape, apple, unsweetened orange, grapefruit, pineapple and exotic fruit juices may be drunk in moderation (e.g. 5 fl oz [125 ml] per day).

See recipes for delicious low-calorie drinks on pages 285–8.

Sauces and dressings

Sauces made without fat, and with low-fat skimmed milk from the daily allowance, may be eaten in moderation. Gravy made with gravy powder, but not granules, may also be served with main courses. (A special recipe for the gravy connoisseur is on page 284.) Vegemite or Bovril may be used freely to add flavour to cooking and on bread. For salads select any of the fat-free dressings (see recipes) and occasionally you can have the seafood dressing or reduced-oil salad dressing where stated, according to the menu selected. Soy and Worcestershire sauce, lemon juice or vinegar may be consumed freely.

Part 4: Daily nutritional requirements

In selecting your menus, each day try to incorporate the following minimum quantities:

6 oz (150 g) protein food (fish, poultry, meat, cottage cheese, baked beans).
12 oz (300 g) vegetables (including salad).
12 oz (300 g) fresh fruit, including fruit juice.
6 oz (150 g) carbohydrate (bread, cereals, potatoes, rice, pasta).
10 fl oz (250 ml) skimmed or semi-skimmed milk.

I would also suggest that one multivitamin tablet be taken daily to make doubly sure that you are getting all the vitamins you need.

Part 5: The forbidden list

Unless they have been included as ingredients in the recipes, these foods are strictly forbidden whilst following the diet (some exceptions are made for vegetarians). Some will be reintroduced for the maintenance programme.

Butter, margarine, Flora, Gold, Gold Lowest, Delight, Outline, or any similar products

Cream, soured cream, whole milk, Gold Top, etc.

Lard, oil (all kinds), dripping, suet, etc.

Milk puddings of any kind except Diet Rice Pudding (see recipe, pages 278–9)

Fried foods of any kind except dry-fried

Fat or skin from all meats, poultry, etc.

All cheese except low-fat cottage cheese unless otherwise stated in the diet menus

Egg yolk (the whites may be eaten freely), except where included in a recipe (although vegetarians should limit their consumption to 3 a week and non-vegetarians to 1 a week)

All nuts except chestnuts

Sunflower seeds

Goose and all fatty meats

Meat products, e.g. Scotch eggs, pork pie, faggots, black pudding, haggis, liver sausage, pâté

All types of sausages and salami

All sauces containing cream or whole milk or eggs, e.g. salad dressing, mayonnaise, French dressing, parsley sauce, cheese sauce, Hollandaise sauce. (Waistline or similar dressings may only be used as stated in the diet menus)

cont.

The forbidden list cont.

Cakes, sweet biscuits, pastries (including savoury pastries), sponge puddings, etc.

Chocolate, toffees, fudge, caramel, butterscotch

Savoury biscuits and crispbreads (except Ryvita)

Lemon curd

Marzipan

Cocoa and cocoa products, Horlicks, except very low-fat brands

Crisps, including low-fat crisps

Cream soups

Avocado pears

Yorkshire pudding

Egg products, e.g. quiches, egg custard, pancakes etc.

Ice cream made with real cream (e.g. Cornish)

Part 6: The binge corrector menu

Inevitably there will be occasions when you are invited to eat food which is forbidden on this diet. It could be a restaurant dinner, a formal occasion such as a wedding, or just a plain, simple party where the buffet offers a high-fat menu. Buffets are the worst – definitely. The slimmer finds it almost impossible to control her or himself once (s)he has 'just tried one of these – one won't do any harm'. Yes, it will happen and when you've done it you'll wish you hadn't and want to know what you can do to correct it.

The Binge Corrector Diet detailed below *is only to be used for one day maximum* to undo the harm you have done on such an occasion and only when you have seriously over-indulged. An *occasional* indiscretion can be corrected simply by returning strictly to the diet the next day. If you use the Binge Corrector Diet too often you will completely ruin your metabolic rate and will find the proper diet less effective.

Breakfast
Large wedge of melon.

Lunch
Slimmers' cup-a-soup.
Diet yogurt.

cont.

The binge corrector menu cont.

Dinner

Large salad of lettuce, cucumber, tomato, sliced
   mushrooms, sliced onion, grated carrot, cabbage.

4 oz (100 g) baked beans OR 2 oz (50 g) chicken
   breast or 3 oz (75 g) cottage cheese.

Soy sauce.

1 piece fresh fruit.

Supper

6 oz (150 g) tomato juice.

Drinks

4 oz (100 g) skimmed milk for tea and coffee.

Unlimited diet colas, slimline drinks, etc.

9
Recipes

The recipes appear under the following headings:
Breakfasts
Lunches
Dinners
   Starters and Soups
   Main Courses: meat
   Main Courses: poultry
   Main Courses: fish
   Main Courses: vegetarian
   Side Dishes: salads and vegetables
   Desserts
Dressings and sauces
Drinks

Weights and measures
For convenience, the following conversion rates have
been used throughout this recipe section:
1 oz = 25 g
1 fl oz = 25 ml
½ pint = 250 ml

BREAKFASTS

Home-made Muesli

(Serves 1)

½ oz (12.5 g) oats
½ oz (12.5 g) sultanas or ½ banana, sliced
2 teaspoons bran
1 eating apple, grated or chopped
milk from allowance or 3 oz (75 g) natural yogurt

Mix all ingredients together and add honey to taste if required.

Alternatively, mix all ingredients (except banana) the night before and leave to soak in skimmed milk.

Stewed Apricots or Prunes

Soak dried fruit overnight in hot black tea and artificial sweetener to taste. Add a pinch of cinnamon if you wish.

Banana Milk Shake

(Serves 1)

1 medium banana, peeled
4 fl oz (100 ml) semi-skimmed milk (use 2 fl oz [50 ml] from allowance)
5 oz (125 g) diet yogurt – any flavour

Place all the ingredients in a food processor and liquidize. Serve in a tall glass.

Banana and Orange Cocktail

(*Serves 1*)

1 banana, peeled
5 fl oz (125 ml) pure orange juice

Break the banana into small pieces.
Place in a food processor or blender. Whiz until smooth, then add the orange juice. Blend well.
Serve in a tall glass with ice and a twist of orange.

Banana and Sultana Cake

(See page 276)

LUNCHES

Pineapple Boat

(*Serves 2*)

1 medium-sized fresh pineapple
8 oz (200 g) seasonal fruit of your choice
10 oz (250 g) diet yogurt – any flavour
cherry or strawberry to decorate

Divide the pineapple into two halves from top to bottom. Do not cut away the leaves – they add to the decorative look. Cut away flesh with a grapefruit knife and cut this flesh into cubes, removing hard core.
Prepare other fruit – wash and cut into bite-sized

pieces and mix with pineapple. Pile into hollowed-out pineapple halves and dress with yogurt.

Serve chilled and decorate with either a cherry or strawberry.

Prawn and Grapefruit Cocktail

(*Serves 2*)

1 fresh grapefruit
6 oz (150 g) peeled prawns
5 oz (125 g) diet grapefruit yogurt
(natural yogurt can be used if preferred)

Peel grapefruit, removing all pith. Separate into segments and place in a dish.

Sprinkle the fresh prawns on to the grapefruit and dress with yogurt.

Fruit Sundae

(See page 266)

Stilton Pears

(*Serves 4: Maintenance Programme*)

6 ripe pears
juice of 1 lemon
2 oz (50 g) Stilton cheese
8 oz (200 g) Shape soft low-fat cheese
2 tablespoons skimmed milk
salt and pepper
1 oz flaked almonds, baked until brown

Peel pears and cut in half lengthways. Remove core

with the bowl of a spoon and paint lemon juice all over pears to prevent discoloration.

Crush Stilton with a fork and work until creamy, then mix with the Shape soft cheese and skimmed milk until smooth. Season to taste.

With a teaspoon, pile cheese mixture into cavities left by the removal of the cores in the pear halves. Sprinkle browned flaked almonds on top and serve on a bed of lettuce.

Cheese and Strawberry Pears

(Serves 1)

1 large ripe pear
lemon juice
4 oz (100 g) low-fat cottage cheese
1 tablespoon strawberry preserve
8 oz (200 g) strawberries, washed and hulled

Peel, halve and core the pear and brush with lemon juice to prevent discoloration. Chop 3 of the strawberries and mix with the cottage cheese and the strawberry preserve. Place this mixture in the core cavities of the two pear halves. Place the pear halves together in a serving dish and surround them with sliced fresh strawberries.

Keep in a refrigerator until required, but eat within 12 hours.

Summer Delight

(Serves 2)

5 oz (125 g) fruit-flavoured diet yogurt
1 pint (500 ml) jelly, made up with water

4 oz (100 g) plain cottage cheese
8 oz (200 g) fresh fruit of your choice
2 oz (50 g) ice cream (non-Cornish variety)

Spoon alternate layers of yogurt, jelly, cottage cheese, fruit and ice cream into a large sundae glass. Garnish with some extra fruit and serve immediately.

Curried Chicken and Yogurt Salad

(*Serves 1*)

3 oz (75 g) chicken breast, cut into cubes
5 oz (125 g) natural diet yogurt
1 teapoon curry powder
unlimited green salad vegetables

Mix yogurt and curry powder together and stir in the cubes of cooked chicken.

Serve on a bed of fresh green salad vegetables.

Chicken Liver Salad

(*Serves 2*)

6 spring onions, trimmed and chopped
2 tomatoes, quartered
2 ins (5 cm) cucumber, finely chopped
2 rashers back bacon
4 oz (100 g) chicken or duck livers
freshly ground black pepper
½ slice (½ oz/12.5 g) bread

For the dressing

> 1 teaspoon French mustard
> 3 tablespoons lemon juice
> 1 tablespoon orange juice
> 1 tablespoon wine vinegar
> salt and black pepper

Dry-fry the spring onions in a non-stick pan. Mix together with the tomatoes and cucumber in a bowl.

Trim all the fat from the bacon, grill well and chop into small pieces. Wash and trim the livers and dry-fry with black pepper in a non-stick pan. Toast the bread and cut into tiny squares.

Prepare the oil-free dressing by placing all the ingredients in a screw-top jar and shaking well. Pour the dressing over the salad vegetables and toss well.

Arrange the salad in 2 bowls and just before serving add the bacon, livers and toast squares to the centre of each bowl. Serve immediately.

Fruit and Chicken Salad

(Serves 1)

> unlimited amounts of shredded lettuce, chopped
> cucumber and any other green salad
> 1 apple
> 1 pear
> 1 orange
> 1 kiwifruit
> 2 oz (50 g) cooked and chopped chicken breast
> 2 tablespoons plain yogurt
> 1 tablespoon wine vinegar
> 1 clove garlic, crushed
> salt and freshly ground black pepper

Place the lettuce and green salad on a large dinner

plate. Prepare the fruits by peeling, coring and slicing. Lay the slices in a circle on top of the salad vegetables and in the centre put the chopped chicken.

Serve with a dressing made of plain yogurt mixed with wine vinegar, garlic and seasonings.

Seafood Salad

(Serves 2)

4 seafood sticks, chopped
2 oz (50 g) prawns
2 oz (50 g) crab (optional)
Seafood Dressing (see recipes 1 & 2, pages 281–2)
shredded lettuce
tomato quarters
cucumber twists
2 lemon quarters

Mix seafood ingredients and dressing together and place on bed of shredded lettuce. Garnish with tomato quarters, cucumber twists and lemon quarters.

Cheese, Prawn and Asparagus Salad

(Serves 2)

4 oz (100 g) cottage cheese
6 oz (150 g) peeled prawns
4 tablespoons chopped and diced cucumber
freshly ground black pepper
unlimited lettuce or watercress
8 oz (200 g) asparagus tips

184

Mix the cottage cheese, prawns and cucumber together, seasoning to taste with the pepper.

Lay the mixture on a bed of shredded lettuce or watercress and decorate with the asparagus tips.

Kiwifruit and Ham Salad

(Serves 1)

2 oz (50 g) French loaf
1 tablespoon Reduced-oil Dressing (see recipe, page 280)
1 oz (25 g) lean ham
2 kiwifruit, peeled and sliced

Cut the loaf lengthways. Spread the dressing on to the bread. Shred the ham and place on top of the bread. Garnish with the kiwifruit.

Carrot Salad

(Serves 1)

2 large fresh carrots, peeled
1 oz (25 g) sultanas

Grate carrots and mix with the sultanas. Serve with a salad or on a jacket potato.

Orange and Carrot Salad

(Serves 1)

1 large orange
green salad vegetables (e.g. cucumber, chicory, chives cabbage)

185

1 onion, chopped
4 oz (100 g) low-fat cottage cheese
4 oz (100 g) grated carrot
1 oz (25 g) sultanas

Remove peel and pith from orange and slice fresh into rounds. Arrange orange flesh on a bed of chopped green salad vegetables (from the list above) and onion.

Place the cottage cheese in the centre, pile the grated carrot on top and then sprinkle with the sultanas.

Dress with Oil-free Orange and Lemon Vinaigrette (see recipe, page 280).

Bean Salad

(Serves 2)

8 oz (200 g) tin red kidney beans
8 oz (200 g) tin cut green beans
8 oz (200 g) tin chickpeas
8 oz (200 g) tin butter beans
1 Spanish onion, peeled and chopped
4 tomatoes, chopped
cucumber, cut into small pieces
3 sticks celery, washed and finely sliced
3 oz (75 g) sultanas
5 oz (125 g) natural yogurt
salt and freshly gound black pepper

Drain the beans and chickpeas. Mix with the fresh vegetables and sultanas. Mix the yogurt in, and season to taste.

Serve as a meal in itself or with other salad vegetables.

Red Kidney Bean Salad

(*Serves 1*)

8 oz (200 g) red kidney beans, cooked
3 oz (75 g) peas, cooked
4 oz (100 g) potato, cooked and chopped
chopped mint, if available
5 oz (125 g) natural yogurt
green salad vegetables
onion rings, fresh

Mix the beans, peas, potato and mint with the yogurt and serve on a bed of salad vegetables. Decorate with onion rings.

Chinese Apple Salad

(*Serves 1*)

1 red apple, thinly sliced
1 green apple, thinly sliced
1 tablespoon lemon juice
6 oz (150 g) fresh beansprouts
few radishes, sliced
2 sticks celery, sliced
spring onions, sliced
curly lettuce to decorate

For the sweet 'n' sour dressing
1½ tablespoons lemon juice
1 level tablespoon clear honey
few drops soy sauce

In a salad bowl, mix the apples and lemon juice thoroughly, then add the beansprouts, radishes, celery and spring onions. Decorate the edge of the bowl with curly lettuce.

Mix together the three ingredients for the dressing and pour it over the salad; toss well and serve immediately.

Chilli Salad

(Serves 4)

1 green pepper, deseeded and diced
1 red pepper, deseeded and diced
1 lb (400 g) potatoes, peeled, diced and cooked
4 spring onions, finely sliced
2 oz (50 g) mushrooms, washed, trimmed and sliced
7½ oz (200 g) tin kidney beans, drained and washed
few drops Tabasco sauce
¼ teaspoon chilli powder
5 tablespoons natural yogurt

In a large bowl, combine all the prepared fresh vegetables and add the washed kidney beans.

In a separate bowl, mix together the Tabasco sauce, chilli powder, and yogurt, and pour this over the prepared salad. Combine thoroughly and serve.

Coleslaw

(See pages 262–3)

Tomato Galantine

(Serves 2)

14 oz (350 g) tin tomatoes
1 medium-sized onion, finely chopped
1 dessertspoon curry powder
3 oz (75 g) cooked spaghetti, roughly chopped

½ teaspoon sugar
salt and pepper
1 tablespoon seed tapioca, soaked in water for approx.
½ hour (pour off any remaining liquid)

Drain tinned tomatoes really well (this is essential) and then scissor-snip into smallish pieces.

Dry-fry the onion until just soft, add the curry powder and cook for a few minutes to release spices.

Mix *all* the ingredients together, adding the eggs last of all.

Place in a wetted mould if you are turning it out on to a plate.

This dish is best left in a refrigerator for a few days before serving.

Sultana Cake

(See page 277)

Banana and Sultana Cake

(See page 276)

Kim's Cake

(See pages 275–6)

Club Sandwich

(*Serves 1*)

2 oz (50 g) lean bacon, with all fat removed
3 slices light bread (e.g. Nimble or Slimcea)
1 teaspoon reduced-oil salad dressing – any brand
1 teaspoon tomato ketchup

½ teaspoon mustard
1 oz (25 g) cooked chicken
1 tomato
shredded lettuce leaves

Grill the bacon until well cooked and crisp. Toast the bread and spread one slice with reduced-oil salad dressing, the second slice with tomato ketchup and the third with mustard.

Slice the chicken and tomato, and place on the first slice. Next add the toast spread with ketchup (ketchup-side up), then add the bacon followed by shredded lettuce. Top with the remaining slice of toast, (mustard-side down) and press together firmly.

Cut diagonally into four triangles and pierce each one with a cocktail stick to hold the layers together. Arrange each sandwich on its long edge and serve immediately.

Hot Herb Loaf

(*Maintenance Programme*)

1 French loaf
4 oz (100 g) very low-fat spread
1 tablespoon mixed dried herbs
juice of ¼ lemon
black pepper
1 clove fresh garlic, crushed

Cream the very low-fat spread with the herbs, lemon juice and pepper. If you like garlic, add a little now.

Cut the loaf into even, slanting slices about 1 in thick. Spread each slice generously with low-fat spread mixture and reshape loaf. Wrap in foil and bake for 10 minutes in a hot oven (200°C, 425°F, Gas Mark 7). Then reduce oven setting to 200°C, 400°F, Gas Mark 6 and open the foil so that the bread browns and crisps. This should take a further 5–8 minutes.

(If you wish to avoid the use of any fat, sprinkle the bread slices with herbs, lemon juice and garlic only.)

Tuna Loaf

(Serves 4)

2 medium-sized onions, peeled
3 sticks celery, washed and trimmed
7 oz (175 g) tuna in brine
2 oz (50 g) fresh breadcrumbs
1½ oz (37.5 g) skimmed milk powder, e.g. Marvel
1 tablespoon tomato purée
2 teaspoon Worcestershire sauce
1 small egg
salt and pepper

Mince or grate the onions and the celery. Drain the tuna and flake the flesh into a bowl. Add all the other ingredients, mix, and season well. Place the mixture in a 1 1b (400 g) non-stick loaf tin and press down carefully. Bake at 180°C, 350°C, or Gas Mark 4 for 1 hour.

Turn out and serve hot or cold with vegetables or salad.

Oat and Cheese Loaf

(See page 260)

Fresh Vegetable Soup

(Serves 4)

2 large carrots, peeled and chopped
1 large potato, peeled and chopped
4 oz (100 g) cabbage, shredded
2 oz (50 g) peas
2 oz (50 g) sweetcorn (optional)
1 large onion, chopped
2 pints (1 litre) water
1 vegetable stock cube
freshly ground black pepper

Place all the vegetables in a large pan with the water. Cover and bring to the boil. Add the stock cube and simmer for 1 hour. Add a generous sprinkling of black pepper to taste. Allow to cool, then place in a food processor or liquidizer on high speed for 15 seconds.

Store in the refrigerator until needed. Deep-freeze any surplus to requirements.

This thick soup is a quick and economical dish that is high in nutrition and low in fat.

Mixed Vegetable Soup

(Serves 8–10)

8 oz (200 g) old but firm potatoes
8 oz (200 g) carrots
8 oz (200 g) onions
8 oz (200 g) leeks
3–4 sticks celery
3½–4½ pints (2–2.5 litres) chicken stock

salt and freshly ground black pepper
chopped fresh parsley or chives to garnish

Peel the potatoes, carrots and onions. Wash and trim the leeks and celery. Grate the potatoes and carrots and finely slice the onions, leeks and celery. (A food processor or mixer with grating and slicing attachments is ideal for this.)

Place the vegetables in a large pan with the chicken stock. Season with salt and freshly ground black pepper. Bring to the boil, cover and simmer gently for 20–30 minutes until all the vegetables are tender. If you prefer a smooth soup, purée the vegetables in a food processor or liquidizer or through a vegetable mill.

Add more stock to thin the soup if necessary. Check the seasoning, reheat and pour into a hot soup tureen. Sprinkle the chopped fresh parsley or chives over the top before serving. Serve hot.

Fish Chowder

(Serves 4)

1 lb (400 g) white fish
1 pint (500 ml) fish stock
1 onion, chopped
1 lb (400 g) small new potatoes
2 large carrots, chopped
4 oz (100 g) mushrooms
4 oz (100 g) baby sweetcorn
2 teaspoons mustard
½ pint (250 ml) skimmed milk
parsley
freshly ground black pepper

193

Poach the fish in the fish stock. Drain, but save the stock. Flake the fish and discard bones and skin.

Dry-fry the onion. Place it and all the other ingredients, excluding the flaked fish, into the fish stock. Simmer until the potatoes are cooked. Add the fish and then serve.

Jacket Potato with Chopped Vegetables

(Serves 1)

½ green and ½ red pepper, deseeded and chopped
1 oz (25 g) tinned sweetcorn
½ onion, chopped
2 mushrooms, chopped
1 oz (25 g) cucumber, chopped
2 tablespoons natural yogurt
salt and freshly ground black pepper
1 cooked jacket potato, halved and opened

Mix the first seven ingredients together and pile on to the two halves of the jacket potato. Serve immediately.

Jacket Potato with Barbecue Topping

(Serves 1)

1 teaspoon Worcestershire sauce
1 tablespoon brown sauce
1 tablespoon tomato ketchup
1 tablespoon mushroom sauce
3 oz (75 g) cooked prawns or chicken if desired
1 cooked jacket potato

Heat the sauces in a small non-stick saucepan. Add prawns or chicken if desired and heat thoroughly.

Serve on the jacket potato.

Jacket Potato with Chicken and Peppers

(Serves 1)

2 oz (50 g) cooked chicken flesh
¼ red and ¼ green pepper, deseeded and chopped
1 tablespoon natural yogurt
1 tablespoon reduced-oil salad dressing
salt and freshly ground black pepper
1 cooked jacket potato

Mix the first five ingredients together and add the contents of the jacket potato.

Pile back into the 'jacket' and reheat in the oven for 5 minutes.

Jacket Potato with Prawns and Sweetcorn

(Serves 1)

2 oz (50 g) prawns
2 oz (50 g) tinned sweetcorn
1 tablespoon reduced-oil salad dressing
1 tablespoon tomato ketchup
salt and freshly ground black pepper to taste
1 cooked jacket potato, halved and opened

Mix the first five ingredients together and pile on to the two halves of the jacket potato. Serve immediately.

Jacket Potato with Chilli Bacon

(*Serves 1*)

1 oz (25 g) lean bacon, chopped
1 small onion, chopped
4 mushrooms, washed and chopped
2 tablespoons chilli sauce
1 cooked jacket potato, halved and opened

Dry-fry the bacon, onion and mushrooms in a non-stick frying pan. When cooked, add the chilli sauce and mix well.

Pile on to the two halves of the jacket potato. Serve immediately.

Potato Madras

(*Serves 2*)

1¼ lbs (500 g) potatoes, peeled and diced small
1 large onion, sliced
8 oz (200 g) frozen sweetcorn
1 oz (25 g) lentils, pre-soaked
14 oz (350 g) tin tomatoes
4 teaspoons curry powder
4 tablespoons vegetable stock
salt and pepper

Dry-fry the potatoes and onion in a large non-stick frying pan. Add all the remaining ingredients; stir well and season. Cover and cook for 15–20 minutes, stirring occasionally.

Serve with 4 oz (100 g) natural yogurt mixed with chopped cucumber.

Stuffed Pepper

(Serves 1)

1 pepper, red or green
1 oz (25 g) [dry weight] brown rice
1 teaspoon mixed herbs
1 teaspoon sweetcorn
1 teaspoon peas
1 teaspoon mushrooms, chopped
½ medium-sized onion, chopped
salt and freshly ground black pepper

Wash the pepper; remove the top and scoop out the seeds.

Boil the rice with the herbs until the rice is tender. Mix the rice and the other vegetables together, season and pile into the pepper. Place on a baking tray in a moderate oven (160°C, 325°F, Gas Mark 3) for 20 minutes.

Serve with other vegetables if desired.

Tofu Burgers

(See page 261)

Oriental Stir-fry

(Serves 4)

12 oz (300 g) potatoes, peeled, grated and well rinsed
6 oz (150 g) frozen sweetcorn
1 large red pepper, deseeded and diced
6 oz (150 g) cauliflower florets
6 oz (150 g) mushrooms, washed and sliced
6 oz (150 g) beansprouts

3 tablespoons soy sauce
3 tablespoons Worcestershire sauce

For the topping
2 tablespoons Parmesan cheese

Dry-fry the potato in a non-stick frying pan for 2 minutes.

Add sweetcorn, diced pepper and cauliflower florets to the pan and fry for 5 minutes. Add remaining ingredients and fry for a further 2 minutes.

Serve immediately with half a tablespoon grated Parmesan cheese sprinkled over each serving.

Baked Stuffed Apple

(See page 279)

DINNERS

Starters and soups

Crudités

Wash, trim and cut into sticks or sprigs of raw vegetables such as cucumber, carrots, celery, green and red peppers and cauliflower. Serve with Garlic or Mint Yogurt Dip (see recipe below).

Garlic or Mint Yogurt Dip

5 oz (125 g) low-fat natural yogurt
1 clove garlic, finely chopped, or 2 sprigs fresh mint,

finely chopped
4 oz (100 g) cottage cheese

Mix the yogurt, garlic (or mint) and cottage cheese together. Serve in a small dish, accompanied by Crudités (see recipe opposite).

Orange and Grapefruit Cocktail

(*Serves 2*)

1 large orange
1 grapefruit

Remove all peel and pith from both fruits. Work the segments from core with a sharp knife and arrange in two dishes. Squeeze as much juice as possible on to the fruit from the peel and core.
  Serve chilled.

Grilled Grapefruit

(*Serves 2*)

1 grapefruit
2 tablespoons sweet sherry
2 teaspoons brown sugar

Cut the grapefruit in half. Remove core and membranes between segments with a grapefruit knife. Pour the sherry over the flesh, and sprinkle the brown sugar on top. Place under a hot grill until sugar is glazed.
  Serve hot.

Melon and Prawn Salad

(Serves 2)

1 melon
4 oz (100 g) peeled, cooked prawns

Halve the melon and remove seeds. Scoop out flesh of melon with a ball-scoop. Mix the melon balls carefully with the prawns, and replace in empty melon shells. Serve chilled.

Pair of Pears

(Serves 1)

1 ripe pear
lemon juice
4 oz (100 g) low-fat cottage cheese
shredded lettuce

Peel, halve lengthways and core the ripe pear, then paint with lemon juice to prevent discoloration. Fill cavities with low-fat cottage cheese and serve on a bed of shredded lettuce.

French Tomatoes

French tomatoes are so called because in the traditional recipe Gervais cream cheese is used in place of the low-fat cottage cheese.

8 tomatoes
salt and pepper
6 oz (150 g) low-fat cottage cheese

small bunch of fresh chives or spring onion tops or
parsley, finely chopped
Oil-free Vinaigrette Dressing (see recipe, page 280)
watercress to garnish

Scald and skin the tomatoes by placing them in a
bowl, pouring boiling water over them and counting
to fifteen before pouring off the hot water and replac-
ing it with cold. The skin then comes off easily.

Cut a slice from the non-stalk end of each tomato
and reserve slices. Hold tomato in the palm of your
hand and remove seeds with the handle of a teaspoon, then remove the core with the bowl of the
spoon. Drain the hollowed-out tomato and season
lightly inside each one with salt.

Soften cheese with a fork and when soft add most
of the finely chopped chives, spring onion tops or
parsley and season well. Fill the tomatoes with the
cheese mixture, using a small teaspoon, until the
mixture is above the rim of each tomato. Replace
their top slices on the slant and arrange tomatoes in
a serving dish.

Make dressing (see recipe, page 280) and spoon
it over the tomatoes, saving some to add just before
serving. Chill tomatoes for up to 2 hours. Before
serving, garnish with watercress and sprinkle
remaining chives and dressing over tomatoes.

Melon Salad

(Serves 4)

1 honeydew melon
1 lb (400 g) tomatoes
1 large cucumber

salt
1 tablespoon parsley
Oil-free Vinaigrette Dressing (see recipe, page 280)
1 heaped teaspoon mint and chives (chopped)

Cut the melon in half, remove the seeds and scoop out the flesh; a curved grapefruit knife is useful for this, if you have one. Cut the flesh into cubes.

Skin and quarter the tomatoes, squeeze out the seeds and remove the core; cut quarters again if the tomatoes are large.

Peel the cucumber, cut into small cubes about the same size as the melon cubes. Sprinkle with salt, cover with a plate and stand for 30 minutes. Drain away any liquid and rinse cubes in cold water.

Mix the fruit and vegetables together in a deep bowl. Pour the dressing over them; cover and chill for 2–3 hours. Just before serving, mix in the herbs.

As the salad makes a lot of juice it should be eaten with a spoon. A Hot Herb Loaf (see recipe, pages 190–1) goes well with melon salad.

Garlic Mushrooms

(*Serves 4*)

1 lb (400 g) button mushrooms
3 cloves fresh garlic
½ pint (250 ml) chicken stock
salt and pepper

Wash mushrooms and drain. Peel and finely slice the garlic cloves. Heat chicken stock with garlic. Boil for 5 minutes on gentle heat, then add mushrooms and simmer in a covered saucepan for a further 7 minutes. Season to taste before serving.

Serve in soup dishes and eat with a spoon.

Ratatouille

(Serves 2)

8 oz (200 g) courgettes
2 aubergines
2 small onions, finely sliced into rings
1 large green pepper
15 oz (375 g) tin tomatoes
2 cloves garlic, chopped (optional)
2 bay leaves
salt and freshly ground black pepper

Slice the courgettes and aubergines. Halve the pepper, remove core and seeds, and cut into fine strips.

Place the tinned tomatoes in a large saucepan and add all the other ingredients. Bring to the boil and skim any sediment if necessary. Cover and simmer for about 20 minutes or until all vegetables are tender. If there is too much liquid remaining, reduce this by boiling briskly for a few minutes with the lid removed.

NB Ratatouille can be used as a main course if accompanied by a chicken joint or 8 oz (200 g) (cooked weight) white fish.

Mixed Vegetable Soup

(See pages 192–3)

Creamy Vegetable Soup

(Serves 4)

1¼ lbs (500 g) potatoes, peeled
8 oz (200 g) carrots, washed and trimmed
2 leeks, washed and trimmed
2 sticks celery, washed and trimmed
2½ pints (1.25 litres) vegetable stock
salt and pepper
2 oz (50 g) skimmed milk powder
1 oz (25 g) cornflour
chopped parsley for garnish

Dice the potatoes and carrots and finely chop the leeks and celery. Place these vegetables in a saucepan with the stock. Season, cover and simmer for 20–30 minutes.

Blend the skimmed milk powder and cornflour with a little cold water and stir into the soup. Bring to the boil and simmer for 5 minutes, stirring all the time.

Garnish with chopped parsley.

Fresh Vegetable Soup

(See page 192)

Leek and Potato Soup

(Serves 4)

3 large leeks, trimmed, cleaned and chopped
2 large potatoes, peeled and chopped
1¾ pints (875 ml) vegetable stock
salt and pepper

Simmer the vegetables in the stock until tender. Liquidize in a food processor and season to taste. This recipe may be reheated if not served immediately.

Butter Bean and Carrot Soup

(Serves 4)

4 oz (100 g) dry butter beans, soaked, cooked and drained
8 oz (200 g) carrots, peeled and sliced
1 small onion, sliced
1½ pints (750 ml) vegetable stock
salt and pepper
1 tablespoon chopped coriander or parsley for garnish

Reserve some of the beans and simmer the remainder of them with the carrots and onions in the stock until tender. Liquidize in a food processor. Return the liquidized vegetables to the saucepan, season, add reserved beans and heat through. Garnish with chopped herb.

Creamy Mushroom Soup

(Serves 4)

2 oz (50 g) onion, chopped
4 oz (100 g) potato, scrubbed and diced
½ pint (250 ml) vegetable or chicken stock
10 oz (250 g) mushrooms, peeled and chopped
½ teaspoon dried thyme
¾ pint (375 ml) skimmed milk
1 bay leaf
freshly ground black pepper to season

Cook the onion and potato gently in the stock for a little while, then add the mushrooms, thyme, milk and bay leaf. Bring to the boil. Reduce heat to a simmer and cook for 25 minutes.

Remove bay leaf. Liquidize, reheat and season to taste. Serve garnished with chopped parsley or chives.

Curried Potato and Parsnip Soup

(Serves 4)

1 onion, chopped
1 large potato, chopped
8 oz (200 g) parsnips, chopped
1 teaspoon curry paste
1 pint (500 ml) vegetable stock
salt and pepper to taste
1 fl oz (25 ml) skimmed milk
1 teaspoon dried parsley

Place the onion, potato, parsnips, curry paste, stock and seasoning in a non-stick pan and bring to the boil. Cover and simmer for 20 minutes or until tender.

Liquidize in a food processor. Return the mixture to the pan and add milk and parsley. Heat through gently and serve.

Curried Courgette Soup

(Serves 6)

1 lb (400 g) courgettes, chopped
1 onion, chopped

1 teaspoon curry powder to taste
1¾ pints (875 ml) vegetable stock
salt and pepper
4 tablespoons cooked brown rice

Simmer the courgettes, onion, curry powder and stock in a large non-stick covered pan for 15–20 minutes or until tender. Liquidize in a food processor. Wipe the non-stick pan clean, return the liquidized ingredients to the pan and season with salt and pepper. Add the rice and heat through.

Beef and Vegetable Soup

(*Serves 4*)

8 oz (200 g) onions, chopped
2 large beef bones bought from a butcher
1 teaspoon mixed herbs
4 oz (100 g) potatoes, peeled and chopped
8 oz (200 g) carrots, peeled and chopped
15 oz (375 g) tin peas
3 beef stock cubes
salt and freshly ground black pepper

For best results, prepare the beef stock a day in advance. To make the stock, place the chopped onion together with the bones and the mixed herbs in a large saucepan with enough water to cover them. Cover with a lid and boil for 1–2 hours. Remove the bones and allow the stock to cool, then place it in the refrigerator. When the stock is thoroughly chilled, skim off any fat that has solidified on the top. Return to the refrigerator and leave overnight. The stock is now ready for the preparation of the soup.

Place potatoes, carrots, peas and the beef stock in

a large saucepan. Bring to the boil, add the stock cubes and simmer for 30 minutes. Season, and serve hot.

Chicken and Mushroom Soup

(Serves 4)

bones of 1 chicken
2 pints (1 litre) vegetable stock (water from cooking vegetables)
1 chicken stock cube
1 onion, sliced
1 carrot, sliced
1 teaspoon mixed herbs
sprinkling of garlic salt if desired
black pepper to taste
1 bay leaf
6 peppercorns
4 oz (100 g) mushrooms, washed and sliced

Place all ingredients except mushrooms in a large saucepan and cover. Bring to the boil and simmer for approximately 2–3 hours. Taste. If too weak, boil a little faster and remove the saucepan lid until liquid has reduced and it tastes appetizing. Strain away bones, peppercorns, bay leaf and vegetables.

Replace soup in saucepan, add sliced mushrooms, cover and cook for 10 minutes.

Serve piping hot.

Chicken Soup

(Serves 4)

1 chicken carcass or 3 chicken stock cubes
2 pints (1 litre) vegetable stock

1 teaspoon mixed herbs
1 large onion, peeled and finely chopped
2 bay leaves
6 peppercorns
salt and freshly ground black pepper

Place the chicken carcass or stock cubes in a large saucepan with the vegetable stock and all remaining ingredients. Bring to the boil, cover the pan and simmer for 1–1½ hours. Taste for flavouring and add 1 (extra) stock cube if necessary. Strain the soup through a colander to remove all bones, bay leaves and peppercorns.

Store in a refrigerator when cool and use within 2 days. Reheat to serve.

Duck Soup

(Serves 4)

1 duck carcass
2 pints (1 litre) vegetable stock
1 chicken stock cube
1 large onion, peeled and finely chopped
1 clove garlic, crushed
1 teaspoon mixed herbs
2 bay leaves
6 peppercorns
salt

Place the duck carcass in a large saucepan with the vegetable stock. Add the chicken stock cube and all the other ingredients. Bring to the boil, cover the pan and simmer for 1½–2 hours. Taste for flavouring and add another (extra) chicken stock cube if necessary.

209

Strain the soup through a colander to remove all bones, the bay leaves and peppercorns. Allow to cool, then store in a refrigerator. The fat will then separate and rise to the surface. When quite cold, remove all solidified fat from the top of the soup.

Use within 2 days and reheat before serving.

DINNERS

Main Courses: meat

Shepherd's Pie

(Serves 4)

1 lb (400 g) minced beef
½ pint (250 ml) water
1 large onion, finely chopped
1 teaspoon mixed herbs
salt and freshly ground black pepper
1 teaspoon yeast, or beef and vegetable extract, e.g. Marmite, Bovril
1 teaspoon gravy powder
1½ lbs (600 g) potatoes, peeled

Boil mince and water in a saucepan for 5 minutes. Drain mince (retaining the liquid) and place in a covered container until required. Meanwhile, place the liquid in the refrigerator. This will cause any fat to rise to the top and set hard so that it can be removed and discarded.

Replace the skimmed liquid in a saucepan. Add the mince, chopped onion, herbs, salt and pepper, and the yeast or beef extract. Mix gravy powder with a little water and add to the meat mixture. Bring to the boil, stirring continually, and leave to simmer for a further 10 minutes.

Boil the potatoes until soft, then remove most of the water, but not all of it, as the potatoes need to be quite wet for mashing. Mash the potatoes and season well, adding a little skimmed milk if necessary to make a soft consistency.

Place the mince in an oval ovenproof dish and cover with the mashed potatoes. Place under a pre-heated grill to brown the top or in a pre-heated oven (160°C, 325°F, Gas Mark 3) for 10 minutes.

Serve with unlimited vegetables.

Spaghetti Bolognese (1)

(Serves 2)

4 oz (100 g) chicken livers (or lamb's liver)
½ pint (250 ml) beef stock
1 medium-sized onion, sliced
1 clove garlic, chopped, or ½ teaspoon dried minced garlic
3 teaspoons tomato purée
1 rounded dessertspoon plain flour
1 tablespoon sweet sherry
salt and freshly ground black pepper
spaghetti

Sauté the livers in a non-stick frying pan until they have changed colour. Remove from pan.

Add a little stock to the pan. Add the onion, garlic and tomato purée. Stir the flour in and mix well. Add the remaining stock and the sherry and continue to stir until boiling. Simmer for 10 minutes and add the livers, coarsely chopped.

Continue to simmer until sauce becomes thick, approximately 10 minutes. Season to taste and serve on a bed of boiled spaghetti.

NB The spaghetti must be an egg-free variety and boiled in water. Add no butter.

Spaghetti Bolognese (2)

(Serves 4)

1 lb (400 g) lean mince
1 large onion, peeled and finely chopped
16 oz (400 g) tin chopped tomatoes
3 oz (75 g) tin tomato purée
half teaspoon oregano
2 cloves garlic, crushed
freshly ground black pepper
1 beef stock cube
7 oz (175 g) spaghetti (non-egg variety)

Heat a non-stick frying pan and as you do so sprinkle liberally with freshly ground black pepper. Dry-fry the mince until the meat has changed colour and all the fat has liquefied. Separate the mince from the fat by draining through a sieve or colander. Discard the fat and put mince to one side. Wipe out the non-stick frying pan with a paper towel until all fat has been removed.

Replace the pan on the heat and add the onion. Cook slowly until the onion has softened and become slightly brown, then add the drained mince. Add all the other ingredients for the sauce and mix carefully. Cook on a medium heat for 15 minutes ensuring that the meat is thoroughly cooked and flavours absorbed.

212

Meanwhile, dissolve the stock cube in a pan of water and bring to the boil. Add the spaghetti and cook until just soft. Drain the spaghetti through a colander and serve on individual plates adding the bolognese sauce in the centre.

Lasagne

(Serves 4)

For the spicy beef sauce
1 lb (400 g) lean minced beef
1 large onion, chopped
16 oz (400 g) tin chopped tomatoes
1 tablespoon tomato purée
2 tablespoons tomato ketchup or 4 fl oz (100 ml) tomato juice
1 tablespoon brown sauce
½ teaspoon Tabasco sauce
2 level teaspoons chilli powder
2 cloves garlic, crushed, or ½ teaspoon dried garlic

8 oz (200 g) wholemeal lasage sheets

For the topping
5 oz (125 g) low-fat plain yogurt
1 medium-sized egg, beaten

Dry-fry the mince in a non-stick frying pan for 10 minutes, stirring frequently, until the meat changes colour. Place the mince in a sieve or fine colander whilst still hot and drain off all the fat.

Wipe out the frying pan with a piece of kitchen paper and dry-fry the onion until soft and brown. Return the mince to the frying pan with the onion. Add the chopped tomatoes and all the other ingredi-

213

ents for the sauce. Mix well and cover. Cook on a low heat, stirring occasionally, for 45 minutes.

Allowing 2 oz (50 g) [dry weight] wholemeal lasagne sheets per person, layer the beef sauce and the lasagne sheets until they are used up. Make the topping by mixing together the low-fat yogurt and the egg and pour this over the layers in the dish. Place in a hot oven and serve when the topping is bubbly.

Mince and Spaghetti Casserole

(*Serves 4*)

1¼ lbs (500 g) minced beef
½ pint (250 ml) water
2 teaspoons mixed herbs
1 beef stock cube
¼ pint (125 ml) water
freshly ground black pepper
16 oz (400 g) tin spaghetti
1–1½ lbs (400–600 g) potatoes, peeled, cooked and mashed

Boil mince in ½ pint (250 ml) of water for approximately 10 minutes, then drain. Place the minced beef in a casserole dish and sprinkle it with the mixed herbs. Dissolve the beef stock cube with ¼ pint of boiling water and then add this to the mince. Sprinkle with plenty of freshly ground black pepper.

Add the spaghetti to the mince and stir gently. Top with the mashed potato, smooth over with a fork and place in a pre-heated oven (180°C, 350°F, or Gas Mark 4) for 1 hour.

Chilli con Carne

(Serves 4)

16 oz (400 g) lean minced beef
1 large onion, chopped
15 oz (375 g) tin chopped tomatoes
2 bay leaves
1 teaspoon Marmite or Bovril
15 oz (375 g) tin red kidney beans
1 teaspoon chilli powder (adjust this ingredient to your
individual taste)
2 cloves garlic, crushed
freshly ground black pepper

Dry-fry the mince and, when thoroughly cooked, drain through a sieve or colander and discard all fat. Meanwhile, wipe away all fat from the frying pan and then dry-fry the chopped onion. When it is just beginning to turn slightly brown, return the meat to the pan with the onion and add the tomatoes, bay leaves, Marmite or Bovril, kidney beans, chilli powder and garlic. Add liberal amounts of freshly ground black pepper. Add water if the mixture becomes too thick and adjust seasoning as necessary.

Serve on a bed of boiled brown rice.

Spicy Meatballs

(Serves 4)

8 oz (200 g) lamb's or pork liver
8 oz (200 g) lean minced beef
4 oz (100 g) wholemeal breadcrumbs
2 tablespoons tomato purée
1 tablespoon French mustard (preferably wholegrain)
salt and freshly ground black pepper

For the sauce
>   2 carrots, peeled and grated
>   1 onion, grated or finely chopped
>   14 oz (350 g) tin chopped tomatoes
>   1 tablespoon demerara or palm sugar
>   1 tablespoon soy sauce
>   1 tablespoon white wine vinegar or cider vinegar

For the pasta
>   8–12 oz (200–300 g) egg-free tagliatelle or
>   other egg-free pasta

Remove any membrane or veins from the liver. Process in a food processor with the minced beef until the mixture is smooth. Alternatively, chop the liver very finely and mix with the minced beef.

Mix the meat with the wholemeal breadcrumbs, tomato purée and French mustard. Season with salt and freshly ground black pepper. Form into balls the size of a walnut and refrigerate until required.

To make the sauce: Place the carrot and onion in a frying pan with a lid. Add the chopped tomatoes (including their juice), demerara or palm sugar, soy sauce and vinegar. Season lightly, bring to the boil and simmer, uncovered, for 15 minutes.

Add the meatballs, cover and simmer for a further 15 minutes until the meatballs and vegetables are cooked. If the sauce is too thin, remove lid and continue cooking for another 5 minutes or so. If it is too thick, add a little water or beef stock until it has a coating consistency. Check the seasoning.

Meanwhile, put the pasta in a pan of boiling salted water and cook until just tender. Drain well. Arrange on a large serving dish and make a well in the centre.

Spoon the meatballs and sauce into the centre of

the pasta. Serve hot, accompanied with vegetables (e.g. carrots, cauliflower, peas or beans).

Spicy Meat Loaf

(*Serves 4*)

¾ lb (300 g) lean mince
4 oz (100 g) lean boiled bacon
1 large onion, finely chopped
1 tablespoon tomato purée
1½ oz (37.5 g) skimmed milk powder (e.g. Marvel)
1 oz (25 g) porridge oats
½ teaspoon made-up mustard
1 tablespoon chopped parsley, preferably fresh
½ teaspoon dried mixed herbs
freshly ground black pepper
2 tablespoons water
14½ oz (363 g) tin apricot halves

Dry-fry the mince to remove all fat and drain well. Prepare the bacon in a food processor or mincer. Mix the mince, bacon and onion together with the tomato purée, milk powder, oats, mustard, parsley and mixed herbs. Season with freshly ground black pepper and add 2 tablespoons of water. Mix well.

Put the apricot halves dome-side down in a 1 lb (400 g) non-stick loaf tin, then carefully place the meat mixture over them. Press the mixture down gently but firmly. Bake at 190°C, 375°F, or Gas Mark 5 for 50–60 minutes. The meat mixture should shrink from the sides of the tin but still be moist. Turn out the loaf on to a plate and the apricots will be on top.

To improve the appearance of the dish, you may like to arrange additional apricots on top just before serving. This dish may be served hot or cold.

Steak and Kidney Pie

(Serves 4)

8 oz (200 g) lean rump or sirloin steak, cut into cubes
8 oz (200 g) kidneys, cut into bite-sized pieces
2 medium-sized or 1 large onion, chopped
½ pint (250 ml) water
1 wineglass red wine
2 beef stock cubes
1 tablespoon gravy powder (e.g. Bisto)
2 lbs (800 g) potatoes, peeled and boiled
2 tablespoons natural low-fat yogurt
2–3 fl oz (50 ml–75 ml) skimmed milk
salt and pepper

Prepare a non-stick frying pan and brown well the cubes of beef steak and kidneys. Place in a pie dish. Dry-fry the onion until soft and add this to the meat in the pie dish.

Place the water, wine and stock cubes in the pan and bring to the boil. Mix the gravy powder with a little cold water and add to the boiling stock in the pan, stirring continuously. The gravy should be quite thick. Add more gravy powder mixed with a little water as necessary. Pour the gravy over the meat in the pie dish.

Mash the boiled potatoes with the yogurt and sufficient skimmed milk to make the consistency quite soft. Season to taste. Carefully spoon (or pipe) the 'creamed' potato on top of the meat and gravy and ensure that it covers it completely. If you spoon the potato on top, spread it carefully with a fork. Place in a pre-heated oven (180°C, 350°F, Gas Mark 4) for 30–40 minutes, or until crisp and brown on top.

Serve with carrots and other vegetables of your choice. This dish may be accompanied by additional gravy if desired.

Steak Surprise

(*Serves 1*)

4 oz (100 g) rump or sirloin steak
1 clove crushed garlic *or* a sprinkle of dried minced
garlic/garlic granules
1 pinch mixed herbs

Sprinkle garlic and herbs on to meat and work into the flesh on both sides with a steak hammer or a fork. Leave for several hours for the flavour to penetrate the flesh. Heat the grill at full temperature for 5 minutes until it is really hot.

Place steak on grill pan and turn after 1 minute to seal in the juices. Lower the grill rack and continue to cook to your liking – rare, medium rare, etc.

Serve with jacket potato, mushrooms cooked in stock, peas and salad.

Fillet Steaks with Green Peppercorns

(*Serves 4*)

4 × 4 oz (100 g) fillet steaks (or rump steaks or sirloin
steaks)
1 tablespoon green peppercorns in brine
5 fl oz (150 ml) dry white wine
1–2 tablespoons brandy (optional)
3–4 tablespoons low-fat fromage frais or yogurt
salt

chopped fresh parsley for garnish
½ bunch watercress

Trim the steaks, removing all fat. Tie string around the outside of each fillet steak, or use a small meat skewer, to hold each one in a neat shape.

Drain and rinse the green peppercorns in cold water. Place in a pan with the dry white wine and boil rapidly until reduced by half.

Place the steaks on a wire rack in a grill pan and cook under a very hot pre-heated grill for 3–5 minutes on each side, or until cooked the way you like them. Or you could cook them on a pre-heated grillade.

Reboil the sauce, adding the brandy (if used) and any meat juices (but no fat) which may have dropped into the grill pan. Remove from the heat and whisk into it the fromage frais or yogurt. Check the seasoning and add a little salt to taste. Reheat without boiling.

Remove the string or skewers from the steaks and place them on a hot serving dish. Pour the sauce over them and sprinkle chopped fresh parsley on top. Garnish with watercress and serve immediately.

Dijon-style Kidneys

(*Serves 4*)

10–12 lamb's kidneys
6 oz (150 g) mushrooms
salt and freshly ground black pepper
7 fl oz (175 ml) red wine
4 tablespoons beef or lamb stock
1 heaped teaspoon arrowroot

3 oz (75 g) plain, low-fat Quark or yogurt
1½ teaspoons Dijon mustard
chopped fresh parsley to garnish

Skin the kidneys, cut them in half and remove the cores. Soak in cold salted water for 20 minutes. Drain well and dry on kitchen paper.

Wash, trim and slice the mushrooms. Season lightly, then cook gently in the red wine and stock for 7–8 minutes until tender.

Meanwhile, dry-fry the kidneys until tender but still slightly pink in the centre. Place on a hot dish, cover and keep hot.

Mix the arrowroot with a little water, and add to the pan containing the mushrooms, red wine and stock. Bring to the boil, stirring all the time. Whisk in the Quark and the mustard a little at a time. Reheat without boiling. Check the seasoning and add more salt and freshly ground black pepper if necessary.

Add the kidneys to the sauce. Pour into a hot dish and sprinkle chopped fresh parsley over the top just before serving. Serve hot.

Pork with Pear Sauce

(*Serves 4*)

4 lean pork chops or butterfly steak
½–¾ pint (250 ml–375 ml) water (approx.)
16 oz (400 g) tin of pear slices
1 teaspoon cornflour mixed with 2 teaspoons water

Trim any fat from the pork chops or butterfly steak. Place the chops or butterfly steak into a non-stick

221

frying pan and cover with water. Simmer for 5 minutes. Drain away the water and replace it with the juice from the tin of pear slices. Simmer the pork or steak until cooked; remove and keep warm.

Thicken the liquid remaining in the pan with the cornflour mixed with water. Serve the pork or steak with the sauce and pear slices accompanied with vegetables such as broccoli or Brussels sprouts.

DINNERS

Main Courses: poultry

Stir-fried Chicken and Vegetables

(*Serves 4*)

16 oz (400 g) chicken (no skin) coarsely chopped
freshly ground black pepper
2 cloves garlic, peeled and crushed
1 heaped teaspoon grated fresh ginger (optional)
6 oz (150 g) [dry weight] brown rice
1 chicken stock cube
4 sticks celery, washed and finely sliced
2 carrots, peeled and coarsely grated
2 Spanish onions, peeled and coarsely chopped
1 green pepper, washed, deseeded and finely sliced
5 oz (125 g) mushrooms, washed and sliced
15 oz (375 g) tin beansprouts, drained

Pre-heat a large frying pan or wok and liberally sprinkle it with freshly ground black pepper. Add the chopped raw chicken and cook until it changes colour, turning frequently. Add the garlic and ginger

222

(if used) and more pepper as desired. Cover the pan, allow the chicken to cook thoroughly for a further 5 minutes and then put to one side. Meanwhile, boil the brown rice together with the chicken stock cube until just soft.

About 4 minutes prior to serving, replace the frying pan on to a brisk heat. Add the celery, carrot, and onion and stir continuously to ensure vegetables cook lightly and do not burn. Then add the pepper, mushrooms and beansprouts. Do not cover the pan as this would make the vegetables turn soft and mushy. Continue to cook on a brisk heat, tossing continually to ensure that the food becomes evenly hot.

When the rice is cooked, drain without rinsing and place on pre-heated plates. Make a well in the centre of each bed of rice and fill with the stir-fried chicken and vegetables. Serve immediately.

Chicken or Prawn Chop Suey

(Serves 1)

1 chicken joint, skinned and boned, *or* 4 oz (100 g)
prawns, peeled
1 tablespoon vegetable stock
1 large carrot, peeled and coarsely grated
1 large onion, finely sliced
2 sticks celery, finely chopped
1 green pepper, deseeded and sliced
15 oz (375 g) tin beansprouts, drained *or* 15 oz (375 g)
fresh moong beansprouts
salt and pepper to taste
soy sauce

Coarsely slice the chicken, add to the vegetable stock

and cook in a large non-stick frying pan or wok on a moderate heat until it changes colour. Add grated carrot, sliced onion and celery, and stir fry.

Add the sliced green pepper and beansprouts and continue to cook until thoroughly hot. Season to taste.

Serve on a bed of boiled brown rice with soy sauce.

Chinese Chicken

(Serves 1)

6 oz (150 g) chicken, skinned and cut into strips
½ Spanish onion, coarsely chopped
1 teaspoon Schwartz Chinese seasoning
6 tablespoons water
2 tablespoons soy sauce
2 tablespoons lemon juice
4 oz (100 g) cut green beans
3 oz (75 g) cucumber, cut into 2 in (5 cm) lengths
½ red pepper, deseeded and cut into strips
4 oz (100 g) button mushrooms, cut in half
4 oz (100 g) beansprouts
3 oz (75 g) sweetcorn

Dry-fry the chicken and onion in a non-stick frying pan or wok for about 5 minutes. Stir in the Chinese seasoning, water, soy sauce and lemon juice. Bring to the boil. Reduce the heat and add all the other vegetables. Stir thoroughly and cook for approximately 5 minutes.

Serve piping hot on a hot plate.

Chicken Chinese-style

(*Serves 4*)

4 chicken breasts, skinned
1 chicken stock cube mixed in 2 fl oz (50 ml) water
1 tablespoon soy sauce
1 onion, chopped
freshly ground black pepper
2 teaspoons cornflour mixed in 3 tablespoons water
boiled brown rice (prepared in advance)
16 oz (400 g) tin beansprouts, drained

Sauté the chicken breasts in a non-stick frying pan until they change colour. Reduce the heat and add the stock cube mixed in the water, then the soy sauce and onion. Season well with plenty of freshly ground black pepper. Cover with a lid and simmer on a low heat for 15–20 minutes, stirring occasionally.

When the chicken is thoroughly cooked, remove the breasts and place them on a pre-heated serving dish and keep warm.

Add the cornflour mixture to the frying pan and thicken to a creamy consistency. Be careful to keep the heat low as overheating at this stage can cause the sauce to go lumpy. If it thickens too quickly, remove from heat immediately and stir vigorously. Add more water if necessary. When cooked, pour sauce over the chicken breasts ready to serve.

Now mix the cooked rice and beansprouts together in a large bowl. Heat mixture thoroughly by placing it in a large colander and rinsing with plenty of boiling water. This method of reheating prevents overcooking.

Serve with soy sauce and vegetables of your choice.

Tandoori Chicken

(Serves 4)

4 × 6 oz (150 g) chicken breasts, skin removed
1½ tablespoons tandoori powder
½ pint (250 ml) natural yogurt
1 clove garlic, peeled and crushed

Make incisions in the flesh of the chicken. Mix the tandoori powder and yogurt together, and with a pastry brush work the mixture into the incisions in the chicken. Mix the crushed garlic into the remaining mixture and paint this all over the chicken joints. Place in a covered dish and leave to marinate for at least 4 hours, preferably longer, turning occasionally.

Pre-heat your grill at medium heat; place the joints on the baking rack, and cook for approximately 25 minutes, turning frequently and painting them with the remaining marinade at frequent intervals to avoid burning.

Serve with green salad and boiled brown rice.

Chicken Curry

(Serves 2)

2 chicken joints with all fat and skin removed
15 oz (375 g) tin tomatoes
1 bay leaf
1 eating apple, cored and chopped small
2 teaspoons oil-free sweet pickle or Branston pickle
1 teaspoon tomato purée
1 medium-sized onion, finely chopped
1 tablespoon curry powder

Place the chicken joints and all the ingredients in a

saucepan and bring to the boil. Put a lid on the saucepan and cook slowly for about one hour, stirring occasionally and making sure the chicken joints are turned every 15 minutes or so. If the mixture is too thin, remove the lid and cook on a slightly higher heat until the sauce reduces and thickens.

Serve on a bed of boiled brown rice.

Barbecued Chicken Kebabs

(*Serves 2*)

For the kebabs
2 large chicken joints, preferably breasts, boned and with all fat and skin removed
2 medium-sized onions, peeled and cut into quarters
1 green pepper and 1 red pepper with core and seeds removed, cut into bite-sized squares
6 oz (150 g) mushrooms, washed but left whole
8 bay leaves

For the barbecue sauce
2 tablespoons tomato ketchup
2 tablespoons brown sauce
2 tablespoons mushroom sauce (optional)
2 tablespoons wine vinegar

Cut the chicken flesh into cubes large enough to be placed on a skewer. Thread on to two skewers alternately with bite-sized pieces of onion, green and red peppers and mushrooms, placing a bay leaf on the skewer at intervals to add flavour.

Mix all the sauce ingredients together and brush on to the chicken and vegetables on the skewers. If you have time, brush the sauce on a couple of hours before cooking, as this will add greatly to the flavour.

227

Place the skewers under the grill and cook under a moderate heat, turning frequently to avoid burning. Continue to baste with the sauce mixture to maintain the moisture. Use no fat.

Serve on a bed of boiled brown rice and grilled fresh tomatoes.

Spaghetti Chicken

(Serves 4)

For the sauce
1½ lbs (600 g) chicken breasts, skinned and finely chopped
1 large onion, finely chopped
16 oz (400 g) tin chopped tomatoes
3 oz (75 g) tomato purée
1 jar Dolmio Bolognese Sauce
½ teaspoonful oregano
2 cloves garlic, crushed
freshly ground black pepper

For the pasta
1 chicken stock cube
10 oz (250 g) spaghetti (non-egg variety)

Heat a non-stick frying pan and as you do so sprinkle liberally with freshly ground black pepper. Dry-fry the chicken until the meat has changed colour. Remove the chicken and put to one side.

In the frying pan cook the onion slowly until it has softened and become slightly brown, then return the chicken to the pan. Add all other ingredients for the sauce and mix carefully. Cook on a medium heat for 15 minutes, ensuring that the meat is thoroughly cooked and flavours absorbed.

Meanwhile, dissolve the stock cube in a pan of water and bring to the boil. Add the spaghetti and cook until just soft; then drain it through a colander. Serve on individual plates and place the sauce, with the chicken in the centre, on top of the spaghetti.

Chicken Fricassée

(Serves 4)

4 chicken breasts, cooked and coarsely chopped
1 pint (500 ml) skimmed milk (in addition to allowance),
infused with 6 peppercorns
2 bay leaves
2 slices onion
1 chicken stock cube
2 dessertspoons cornflour mixed in 3 tablespoons water
salt and pepper

Infuse the milk and seasonings (bay leaves, onion and stock cube) by bringing to the boil, covering with a lid and leaving for 15–20 minutes.

Strain the milk into another pan and bring almost to boiling point. Remove from the heat, add the slaked cornflour and mix thoroughly. Return to the heat and slowly bring to boiling point, stirring all the time. Season to taste. Add the chopped chicken and continue cooking on a low heat for 5 minutes.

Serve with unlimited vegetables of your choice.

Chicken Veronique

(Serves 4)

1 whole chicken (4 lb) [1.6 kg]
4 sprigs fresh tarragon or 1 teaspoon dried tarragon

salt and freshly ground black pepper
8 oz (200 g) green grapes
½ pint (250 ml) chicken stock
2 tablespoons cornflour
2 fl oz (50 ml) skimmed milk

Place chicken on a rack to keep it away from the fat as it drips away during cooking. Cover with tin foil and cook for 1½ hours at 200°C, 400°F, or Gas Mark 6. Remove foil 30 minutes from end of cooking time.

The grapes must now be peeled and deseeded. If they are difficult to peel, scald them with boiling water for 10 seconds and then drain and place in cold water for 10 seconds. The skin can then be removed easily. Remove the pips. Place the peeled, pipped grapes in an airtight container while you make the sauce.

Sauce
Chicken stock should ideally be made from the giblets which are boiled with an onion, bay leaf and peppercorns in water for 30 minutes and allowed to cool. Then remove any fat after it has set. A chicken stock cube added to this liquid will strengthen the flavour. If there are no giblets available, make up ½ pint (250 ml) of stock with two chicken stock cubes.

Mix the cornflour with the skimmed milk and carefully add to the stock liquid, stirring continuously. Heat gently and bring to the boil, continuing to stir all the time.

When everything is prepared add the grapes to the chicken sauce which will be light in colour.

Serve chicken either whole or in small joints which can be placed on a bed of sliced onions and potatoes cooked in chicken stock. If the chicken is served whole, serve the sauce separately in a boat. If it is served already jointed, pour the sauce over the completed dish.

Chicken à l'Orange

(Serves 4)

4 chicken breasts
1 wineglass red wine
3 oranges
1 large Spanish onion, chopped
onion salt and white pepper to taste
1–2 tablespoons redcurrant jelly
2 teaspoons cornflour
¼ pint (125 ml) chicken stock

Remove any skin from the chicken breasts and leave to marinate in the red wine for 1 hour. Meanwhile squeeze the juice from the oranges and peel and slice the onion.

Pre-heat a non-stick frying pan and sprinkle with onion salt and white pepper. When the pan is hot, add the chicken pieces (leaving the wine to one side for the moment) and sauté them on a brisk heat until they have changed colour, turning the chicken over to cook both sides. Add the onion or, if there is no room in the pan, dry-fry it in another non-stick frying pan. When the onion has become soft and brown add it to the chicken. Pour into the pan the wine, orange juice and redcurrant jelly. Cover and leave to simmer on a very low heat for 15 minutes or until the chicken is thoroughly cooked.

Meanwhile mix the cornflour with the chicken stock. When the chicken breasts are cooked, remove them from the pan and place on a pre-heated serving dish to keep warm. Into the pan gradually add the chicken stock and cornflour mixture and mix. Slowly bring to the boil, stirring all the time. Taste and adjust the seasoning accordingly.

When ready to serve, pour the orange sauce over the chicken pieces and serve immediately with unlimited potatoes and other vegetables.

Coq au Vin

(*Serves 4*)

3½–4 lb (1.3–1.8 kg) roasting chicken
4 oz (100 g) back bacon, with all fat removed
4 oz (100 g) button onions
7 fl oz (175 ml) red wine (preferably Burgundy)
2 cloves garlic, crushed with ½ teaspoon salt
bouquet garni
¼–½ pint (125–250 ml) chicken stock
salt and pepper
2 dessertspoons cornflour mixed in 3 tablespoons water
chopped parsley for garnish

Joint and skin the chicken and place in a non-stick frying pan. Over a fairly brisk heat, brown the chicken all over and then remove from the pan while other ingredients are prepared. Cut the bacon into strips, approximately 1½ in (3.75 cm) long, and blanch these and the onions by putting them in a pan of cold water, bringing to the boil and draining well.

Put the onions and bacon into the frying pan and cook over a brisk heat until they are brown. Replace the chicken joints and pour the wine over them. Bring to the boil and 'flame' by setting the pan alight

232

with a match. This removes the alcohol from the wine.

Add the crushed garlic, bouquet garni, stock and seasoning. Cover the pan and cook slowly for about 1 hour, or place in a casserole and put in a pre-heated oven (150°C, 325°F, Gas Mark 3).

Test to see that the chicken is tender and that it is thoroughly cooked. Remove the chicken and bouquet garni, put to one side and keep warm. Slowly pour the cornflour paste into the sauce, stirring continuously to keep it smooth. Return to the heat and boil, stirring all the time. Put the chicken pieces back into the casserole and spoon the sauce over them.

Garnish with chopped parsley and serve with French loaf.

DINNERS

Main Courses: fish

Snapper Florentine

(*Serves 1*)

10 oz (250 g) white fish – snapper, trevalli, haddock or cod
lemon juice
5 oz (125 g) natural yogurt
1 lb (400 g) fresh spinach, cooked and chopped, *or* 10 oz (250 g) frozen spinach, thawed and drained
salt and freshly ground black pepper
1 lemon for garnish

Grill the fish on tin foil for 10 minutes, keeping it

moist with lemon juice, or poach for 15–20 minutes in skimmed milk.

Place the yogurt in a saucepan and add the chopped spinach. Heat gently, stirring continuously. Do not boil as the yogurt will curdle. Add salt and black pepper to taste.

Place the spinach mixture on a hot serving dish and arrange the fish on top.

Serve with wedges of lemon.

Fish Pie

(*Serves 4*)

1½ lbs (600 g) cod
1½ lbs (600 g) potatoes, peeled
salt and pepper
2 oz (50 g) low-fat Cheddar (optional for Maintenance dieters only)

Bake, steam or microwave the fish but do not overcook. Season well.

Boil the potatoes until well done and mash with a little water to make a soft consistency. Season well.

Place fish in an ovenproof dish. Flake the flesh, remove the skin, and distribute the fish evenly across the base of the dish. Sprinkle the grated cheese at this point if you are on the Maintenance Diet.

Cover the fish completely with the mashed potatoes and smooth over with a fork. Sprinkle a little cheese on the top if desired.

If the ingredients are still hot just place under a hot grill for a few minutes to brown the top.

Alternatively, the pie can be made well in advance and then warmed through in a pre-heated moderate oven (180°C, 350°F, Gas Mark 4) for 20 minutes, or microwaved on *high* for 5 minutes.

Prawn Chop Suey

(See Chicken or Prawn Chop Suey, pages 223–4)

Fish Curry

(*Serves 2*)

2 pieces frozen haddock
15 oz (375 g) tin tomatoes
1 bay leaf
1 eating apple, cored and chopped small
2 teaspoons oil-free sweet pickle or Branston pickle
1 teaspoon tomato purée
1 medium-sized onion, finely chopped
1 tablespoon curry powder

Place all the ingredients except the fish in a saucepan, and bring to the boil. Put a lid on the saucepan and cook slowly for about 1 hour, stirring occasionally. Approximately 20 minutes before the end of cooking time, add the fish to the saucepan.

If the mixture is too thin, remove the lid and cook on a slightly higher heat until the sauce reduces and thickens towards the end of cooking time.

Serve on a bed of boiled brown rice.

Fish Risotto

(*Serves 4*)

3 frozen haddock fillets
4 tablespoons brown rice

1 onion, chopped
oregano
salt and black pepper
2 oz (50 g) mushrooms, sliced
8 oz (200 g) tin tomatoes
1 glass white wine
2 oz (50 g) frozen peas
1 oz (25 g) low-fat Chedder cheese, grated (optional, for
Maintenance dieters only)

Poach the fish in water until it is cooked. Remove the skin and break the flesh into chunks.

Meanwhile, cook rice in salted water, adding the chopped onion as soon as rice is simmering.

When the rice is half cooked, add the oregano, pepper, mushrooms and tomatoes. Next add the glass of wine and the frozen peas.

Add the fish when almost all the liquid has evaporated.

If you are on the Maintenance Diet, you can sprinkle the risotto with cheese before serving.

For special occasions, you could add green peppers or prawns.

Mussels in White Wine

(*Serves 4*)

4½ lbs (2 kg) mussels
1 small onion, finely chopped
1 clove garlic, crushed, or ½ teaspoon garlic paste
(optional)
a few parsley stalks
1 sprig thyme
5 fl oz (125 ml) dry white wine, or dry cider if preferred

freshly ground black pepper
1–2 tablespoons chopped fresh parsley

Wash the mussels well in several changes of water until they are free of sand and grit. Discard any which are broken or which remain open after being plunged into cold water or given a sharp tap. With a small knife, scrape the barnacles off the shells and remove the beards (the black threads hanging from the mussels).

Place the onion and garlic in a large pan with the parsley stalks, thyme and dry white wine or cider. Cover and simmer gently for about 5 minutes until the onion is nearly tender.

Add the mussels, season with freshly ground black pepper, cover and cook for a further 5–7 minutes over a good heat, shaking the pan occasionally, until all the mussels are open. If the odd mussel remains closed, discard it.

Pile the mussels into a large serving bowl or individual dishes. Pour over them the cooking liquor, discarding the last few spoonfuls if they retain any grit. Sprinkle the mussels with chopped fresh parsley and serve immediately.

Fish Chowder

(See pages 193–4)

DINNERS

Main Courses: Vegetarian

Vegetable Bake

(*Serves 1*)

selection of vegetables, e.g. carrots, parsnips, peas,
cabbage, leeks, onions
1 teaspoon mixed herbs
3 tablespoons packet stuffing mix
4 oz (100 g) mushrooms
6 oz (150 g) potato, cooked
cup of breadcrumbs – preferably wholemeal
½ pint (250 ml) vegetable stock

Cook the selected vegetables, chop them, and place
in layers in a large ovenproof dish. Sprinkle the
mixed herbs and stuffing mix between layers.

Slice the mushrooms and place over the other
vegetables. Then, slice the pre-cooked potato, carefully lay across the top of the dish and sprinkle with
the breadcrumbs. Carefully pour over the vegetable
stock to moisten the contents of the dish.

Bake in a moderate oven (180°C, 350°F, Gas Mark
4) for 20 minutes until piping hot. Alternatively,
reheat in a microwave on *medium* for 7 minutes and
place under a hot grill for 5 minutes to crisp the top.

Vegetable Casserole

(*Serves 1*)

selection of vegetables (approx 1 lb [400 g] in total),
chopped

4 oz (100 g) lentils, pre-soaked
1 teaspoon paprika
pinch of garlic granules
salt and freshly ground black pepper
½ pint (250 ml) water or vegetable stock

Place chopped vegetables and lentils in a casserole and sprinkle with the paprika and garlic granules. Add salt, pepper and stock; cover the casserole.

Place in a moderate oven (180°C, 350°F, Gas Mark 4) and cook for approximately 1 hour or until vegetables are tender.

Alternatively, this dish could be cooked in a microwave for 20–25 minutes on full powder, but use only 3 fl oz (75 ml) water.

Vegetable Chop Suey

(*Serves 1*)

1 tablespoon vegetable stock
1 large carrot, peeled and coarsely grated
3 sticks celery, finely chopped
1 large onion, finely chopped
1 green pepper, deseeded and sliced
15 oz (375 g) tin beansprouts, drained
salt and pepper to taste
soy sauce

Pour a little stock into a non-stick frying pan or wok. Add all ingredients except beansprouts, and stir fry. When the vegetables are hot and partly cooked add the drained beansprouts. Continue to cook for 5 minutes until hot.

Serve on a bed of boiled brown rice, with soy sauce.

Vegetable Kebabs

(Serves 2)

1 green pepper, deseeded and chopped into ¾ in (2 cm)
squares
1 red pepper, deseeded and chopped into ¾ in (2 cm)
squares
1 large Spanish onion, peeled and cut into large pieces,
or 6 oz (150 g) small button onions, peeled
8 oz (200 g) button mushrooms, washed
4 courgettes, coarsely sliced
1 lb (400 g) average-sized fresh tomatoes, sliced across
1 teaspoon thyme
cayenne pepper
2 oz (50 g) Edam or low-fat Cheddar cheese (for
Maintenance dieters only)

Pre-heat oven to 180°C, 350°F, or Gas Mark 4.

Thread vegetable pieces alternately on four skewers to make four kebabs.

Cover a baking sheet with foil and place the kebabs on the foil, sprinkling each kebab with thyme. Wrap the foil around the kebabs to make a parcel and cook for 35 minutes.

Remove from oven. Place on a bed of hot sweetcorn and boiled rice and sprinkle with cayenne pepper to taste. Replace in the oven for 1 minute.

For Maintenance Programme only: Grated Edam or low-fat Cheddar cheese may be sprinkled on to the kebabs at the end of first 35 minutes cooking. Then place serving dish under a pre-heated grill for 2 minutes to melt cheese.

Vegetable Curry

(*Serves 4*)

3 oz (75 g) [dry weight] soya chunks *or*
chopped tofu or tinned vegetable protein
15 oz (375 g) tin tomatoes
1 bay leaf
1 eating apple, chopped
2 teaspoons oil-free sweet pickle or Branston pickle
1 teaspoon tomato purée
1 medium-sized onion, chopped
1 tablespoon curry powder

Soak the soya chunks in 2 cups of boiling water for 10 minutes. Drain.

Place the soya chunks and all other ingredients in a saucepan and bring to the boil. Cover the saucepan and simmer for about 1 hour, stirring occasionally. If the mixture is too thin, remove the lid and cook on a slightly higher heat until the sauce reduces and thickens.

Serve on a bed of boiled brown rice.

Vegetable and Fruit Curry

(*Serves 4*)

1 medium-sized onion, chopped
1 large clove garlic, crushed
1–2 green chillis (according to taste), deseeded and finely chopped
1 in (2.5 cm) piece green ginger, peeled and finely chopped
½ pint (250 ml) vegetable stock
2 teaspoons garam masala

1 teaspoon ground coriander
1 teaspoon ground cumin
8 oz (200 g) green beans
12 oz (300 g) cauliflower florets
1 red pepper, deseeded and finely chopped
salt
2 bananas

Using a non-stick frying pan, dry-fry the chopped onion, garlic, chillis and ginger for 5 minutes on a gentle heat and cover the pan with a lid. Add a little of the vegetable stock if it is too dry.

When the onions are soft, add 2 fl oz (50 ml) of the vegetable stock and then sprinkle the spices over and cook for a further minute, stirring all the while.

Trim the beans and cut into 1 in (2.5 cm) lengths. Add these, the cauliflower and the red pepper to the pan and cook over a moderate heat for 2–3 minutes, stirring continually. Pour in the remaining vegetable stock and season with salt. Cover the pan and cook gently for 10 minutes.

Peel and slice the bananas and add to the pan. Cook for a further 10 minutes or until the vegetables are tender.

Serve with boiled brown rice and a bowl of yogurt mixed with chopped cucumber and a little mint sauce.

Vegetable Chilli

(*Serves 4*)

15 oz (375 g) tin tomatoes
1 bay leaf
1 eating apple, chopped
2 teaspoons oil-free sweet pickle or Branston pickle

1 teaspoon tomato purée
1 medium-sized onion, chopped
4 oz (100 g) broad beans
4 oz (100 g) peas
4 oz (100 g) carrots, peeled and chopped
4 oz (100 g) potatoes, peeled and chopped
8 oz (200 g) tin baked beans or red kidney beans
1 teaspoon chilli powder   } adjust seasoning
3 chillis   } to individual
1 teaspoon garlic granules   } taste
4 fl oz (100 ml) vegetable stock

Place all ingredients in a saucepan and cover. Simmer for 1 hour, stirring occasionally. Remove lid and continue to cook until of a thick consistency, raising the heat if necessary to reduce the liquid. Serve on a bed of boiled brown rice.

Vegetarian Goulash

(*Serves 2*)

3 oz (75 g) soya chunks
1 large onion, chopped
3 oz (75 g) carrots, sliced
3 oz (75 g) potato cut into small chunks
15 oz (375 g) tin tomatoes
½ pint (250 ml) vegetable stock
1 red pepper, deseeded and chopped
2 bay leaves
2 teaspoons paprika
3 tablespoons natural yogurt
salt and black pepper to taste

Soak the soya chunks in 2 cupfuls of boiling water for 10 minutes and drain.

Place all the ingredients except the yogurt in a saucepan. Bring to the boil, cover and simmer for about 1 hour. Stir in the yogurt and season to taste. Serve with boiled brown rice or wholewheat pasta.

Vegetarian Shepherd's Pie

(Serves 4)

3 oz (75 g) [dry weight] soya savoury mince
1 large onion, finely sliced
15 oz (375 g) tin tomatoes, finely chopped
1 teaspoon mixed herbs
salt and freshly ground black pepper
1 teaspoon yeast extract
4 fl oz (100 ml) vegetable stock
1 tablespoon gravy powder mixed in a little water
1½ lbs (600 g) cooked potatoes, mashed (with water only)

Add soya savoury mince to 2 cups of boiling water and leave to soak for 10 minutes. Drain.

Place the soya mince, onion, tomatoes, herbs, seasoning, yeast extract and vegetable stock in a saucepan. Bring to the boil and simmer for 20 minutes. Add the gravy powder mixed with water and stir until mixture thickens. Simmer uncovered for a further 5 minutes.

Place the mince mixture in an oval ovenproof dish and cover with the mashed potatoes. Place under a pre-heated grill to brown the top, or in a pre-heated oven (160°C, 325°F, Gas Mark 3) for 10 minutes.

Serve with unlimited vegetables.

Vegetarian Chilli con 'Carne'

(Serves 4)

3 oz (75 g) [dry weight] soya savoury mince
15 oz (375 g) tin tomatoes
2 bay leaves
1 large onion, chopped
1 teaspoon yeast extract
15 oz (375 g) tin red kidney beans
1 teaspoon chilli powder (adjust this ingredient to your
individual taste)
1 teaspoon garlic granules (optional)

Add 2 cups of boiling water to soya mince and leave
to soak for 10 minutes.

Place all ingredients in a saucepan, cover and cook
for 30 minutes. Remove lid and continue cooking
until it reaches a fairly thick consistency.

Serve with boiled brown rice.

Vegetarian Spaghetti Bolognese

(Serves 4)

3 oz (75 g) [dry weight] soya mince
3 oz (75 g) mushrooms
15 oz (375 g) tin tomatoes
½ green pepper, deseeded and finely chopped
1 teaspoon yeast extract
1 teaspoon oregano
2 cloves garlic, chopped
1 tablespoon gravy powder
egg-free spaghetti

Pre-soak the soya mince in 2 cups of boiling water
and leave to stand for 10 minutes. Drain.

Place soya mince, mushrooms, tomatoes, pepper, yeast extract, oregano and garlic in a saucepan; cover and simmer for 20 minutes. Mix gravy powder with a little cold water and mix into the sauce mixture.

Boil spaghetti for 10–20 minutes until tender. Drain and place in a serving dish. Pour sauce on top.

Tricolour Pasta

(Serves 3–4 people)

1 tablespoon olive oil
1 onion, cut in half and shredded
8 oz (200 g) courgettes, topped and tailed and thinly cut lengthwise – discard the first slice, then cut in 1½ in (4 cm) long pieces across
1 red pepper, cut into 1½ in (4 cm) long strips
3 oz (75 g) petits pois
8 oz (200 g) tricolour pasta spirals
¾ pint (375 ml) water
1 vegetable stock cube
14 oz (350 g) tomatoes
2 teaspoons freshly chopped *or* 1 teaspoon dry marjoram
salt and freshly ground black pepper

To serve
2 oz (50 g) strong cheese, grated

Heat the olive oil and fry the onion and courgettes for 3 minutes. Add the red pepper, peas, pasta, water and stock cube, tomatoes and marjoram. Bring back to the boil, cover, and simmer for 20 minutes.

Season, then leave the mixture to stand for 5 minutes before serving with grated cheese and crisp salad.

Lyonnaise Potatoes

(*Serves 2–4*)

1 lb (400 g) potatoes scrubbed but not peeled
2 large Spanish onions
garlic granules
¼–½ pint (125–250 ml) skimmed milk
chopped parsley

Slice the potatoes and onions. Place in layers in a casserole dish, sprinkling a few garlic granules between layers. Pour over the vegetables enough skimmed milk almost to reach the top layer. Cover and cook in a moderately hot oven (200°C, 400°F, Gas Mark 6) for ¾–1 hour or until tender.

Garnish with chopped parsley.

Hummus with Crudités

(*Serves 2*)

For the hummus

4 oz (100 g) chickpeas, pre-soaked in cold water
overnight
7 tablespoons skimmed milk in addition to allowance
1 tablespoon lemon juice
½ teaspoon mild chilli powder
¼ teaspoon garlic granules
¼ teaspoon ground white pepper
salt
2 tablespoons natural yogurt

For the crudités

red pepper ⎫
cucumber ⎬ all cut into sticks
celery ⎭
cauliflower florets – for dipping

Drain the chickpeas and place in a saucepan. Cover with fresh water and bring to the boil. Reduce the heat, cover and simmer gently for 2–2¼ hours until chickpeas are soft. Drain.

Place chickpeas, skimmed milk and lemon juice in a food processor or liquidizer and blend on high speed until mixture is pale and smooth. Stir in to this the chilli powder, garlic granules, white pepper, salt and yogurt.

Spoon into a serving dish and chill before serving.

Serve with raw vegetable sticks and cauliflower florets.

Bean Salad

(See page 186)

Three Bean Salad

(*Serves 4*)

15 oz (375 g) tin red kidney beans, drained and washed
15 oz (375 g) tin haricot beans, drained and washed
8 oz (200 g) tin butter beans, drained and washed
1 cucumber, finely chopped
3 tomatoes, finely chopped
4 sticks celery, finely sliced
8 spring onions, finely sliced
1 red or green pepper, finely chopped
1 Spanish onion, finely chopped
sprinkling of oregano and sage
salt and freshly ground black pepper

Mix all ingredients together in a large bowl. Serve chilled with French bread, garlic bread or Hot Herb

Loaf (see recipe, pages 190–1) if you are on the Maintenance Programme.

Spiced Bean Casserole

(*Serves 2*)

2 oz (50 g) chopped onion
8 oz (200 g) tin tomatoes
¾ teaspoon mild chilli powder
½ tablespoon tomato purée
1 oz (25 g) wholemeal flour
¼ pint (125 ml) beef-flavoured stock
½ teaspoon garlic granules
pinch of salt
4 oz (100 g) courgettes, sliced
6 oz (150 g) red and green peppers, sliced
8 oz (200 g) tin red kidney beans, washed and drained
8 oz (200 g) tin haricot beans, drained
4 oz (100 g) sweetcorn

Dry-fry the onion in a non-stick frying pan until soft. Add tinned tomatoes, mild chilli powder, tomato purée and wholemeal flour and mix well.

Gradually add the beef-flavoured stock together with the garlic granules, salt, sliced courgettes and peppers. Add the drained beans and sweetcorn and bring to the boil. Cover and simmer for 10–12 minutes or until the vegetables are tender.

Serve with mashed potatoes or boiled rice.

Blackeye Bean Casserole

(*Serves 2*)

2 oz (50 g) blackeye beans
2 oz (50 g) onion, diced

6 oz (150 g) mushrooms, sliced
4 oz (100 g) celery, cut into thin strips
3 oz (75 g) carrots, cut into thin strips
2 oz (50 g) water chestnuts, thinly sliced
½ teaspoon, chilli powder
ginger
1 clove garlic, chopped
½ oz (12.5 g) cornflour
1 tablespoon soy sauce
¼ pint (125 ml) vegetable stock
freshly ground black pepper

Cook the blackeye beans in plenty of water for 30–35 minutes by bringing to the boil and then simmering in a covered pan. Drain the beans.

Gently heat the other vegetables, chilli, ginger and garlic in a little stock for 10 minutes. Mix the cornflour and soy sauce with a little stock and then stir the rest of the stock in. Add this mixture to the vegetables and then add the drained beans. Simmer for 8–10 minutes and season to taste.

Serve on a bed of boiled brown rice.

Chickpea and Fennel Casserole

(Serves 2)

3 oz (75 g) cooked chickpeas
1 oz (25 g) Bulgar wheat
6 oz (150 g) celery, diced
1 dessertspoon crushed fennel seeds
1 clove garlic, crushed
½ pint (250 ml) vegetable stock
6 oz (150 g) whole green beans, chopped
2 tablespoons soy sauce

salt and freshly ground black pepper
2 tablespoons chopped mint, preferably fresh

Cook the chickpeas, wheat, celery, fennel and garlic gently in a little stock for about 5 minutes. Add the remaining ingredients, excluding the mint.

Simmer for 20 minutes and serve with fresh mint and unlimited vegetables.

Chickpea Couscous

(*Serves 4*)

1 tablespoon sunflower or vegetable oil
2 medium carrots, peeled and halved lengthwise and sliced across
1 medium-to-large potato, peeled and chopped
½ cauliflower, cut into florets
8 oz (200 g) courgettes, chunkily chopped
2–3 oz (50–75 g) green beans, cut in half across
1 teaspoon ground coriander
2 vegetable stock cubes
¾ pint (375 ml) water or light stock
¼ pint (125 ml) ready-made tomato sauce
1 medium-sized red pepper, diced
4 oz (100 g) okra, topped and tailed and cut in half across
2 green chillies
1 tablespoon tikka pasta or other marinade paste
14 oz (350 g) tin chickpeas, drained and rinsed
salt and freshly ground black pepper

Heat the oil in a medium-sized saucepan and gently fry the carrots, potato and cauliflower. Stir the mixture from time to time to prevent it sticking to the bottom of the pan. Add the courgettes, green beans and coriander and cook slowly for another 5 minutes.

Add the stock cubes, water or stock, tomato sauce, red pepper, okra, chillies, tikka paste and chickpeas and cook for 20–30 minutes.

Season well with salt and pepper and serve hot on a bed of cooked couscous, quinoa or rice.

Three-layer Millet Bake

(Serves 4)

8 oz (200 g) millet
2 teaspoons bouillon powder or 1½ vegetable stock cubes

For the base
1 tablespoon olive oil
1 onion, peeled and finely chopped
8 oz (200 g) courgettes, chopped
2 cloves garlic, crushed
14 oz (350 g) tin chopped tomatoes
1–2 tablespoons tomato purée
1 teaspoon fresh mixed herbs
2 tablespoons fresh chopped parsley
salt and freshly ground black pepper

For the topping
½ pint (250 ml) plain yogurt
4 oz (100 g) strong Cheddar cheese, grated
good pinch of ground cumin

Place the millet and the bouillon powder or stock cubes in a medium-sized saucepan. Add ¾ pint (375 ml) water, bring the mixture to the boil, cover with a lid and simmer for 20 minutes.

Meanwhile make the base. Heat the oil and fry the onion, courgettes and garlic on a medium heat until tender. Add the tomatoes and tomato purée and boil for 5 minutes. Add the mixed herbs, parsley and seasoning.

To prepare the topping, place the yogurt in a mixing bowl and stir into it the grated cheese and cumin.

Place the tomato mixture in a 2½ pint (1.25–1.5 litre) ovenproof dish, cover with the cooked millet and finish with the yogurt layer. Bake in a pre-heated oven at 190°C, 375°F, Gas Mark 5 for 30 minutes or until the yogurt is set.

Leave to stand for 5 minutes and serve hot with salad.

Mixed Grain and Fresh Coriander Medley

(Serves 4)

½ oz (12.5 g) butter or vegetable margarine
10 oz (250 g) field mushrooms, halved across and sliced
1 rounded teaspoon Marmite
1 tablespoon tamari
4 oz (100 g) couscous
4 oz (100 g) bulgar wheat
4–6 tablespoons fresh chopped coriander
2 beef tomatoes, sliced
2 oz (50 g) mozarella cheese, grated
salt and freshly ground black pepper

Heat the butter or margarine and fry the mushrooms on a medium heat until tender.

Make up some stock by mixing Marmite and tamari with ¾ pint (375 ml) boiling water. Add the stock to the mushrooms, then add the couscous, bulgar wheat and all but 1 tablespoon fresh chopped coriander. Season well.

Place the mixture in a 2½–3 pint (1.25–1.5 litre)

ovenproof dish and top with the sliced tomatoes. Sprinkle the cheese on top of the tomatoes and finish with the remaining fresh coriander. Season with plenty of black pepper and a little salt.

Bake in a pre-heated oven at 200°C, 400°F, or Gas Mark 6 for 20 minutes. Leave to stand for 5 minutes prior to serving.

Stuffed Marrow

(Serves 4)

1 medium-sized marrow, peeled, cut in half lengthways and deseeded

For the stuffing
8 oz (200 g) assorted vegetables, chopped
1 oz (25 g) chopped onion
2 cloves garlic, peeled and crushed
2 tablespoons tomato purée
2 teaspoons chopped fresh rosemary *or* 1 teaspoon dried rosemary
salt and freshly ground black pepper
1 vegetable stock cube
4 oz (100 g) long-grain brown rice

Cook the vegetables, onion, garlic, tomato purée and rosemary in a little water seasoned with salt and pepper. Simmer until tender. Leave this mixture for the flavour to develop overnight.

Crumble the vegetable stock cube into a saucepan of boiling salted water, then add the rice and cook until tender. Mix the rice with the vegetable mixture and spoon into the 'well' of the marrow halves.

Wrap the stuffed marrow in foil and bake in the oven at 200°C, 400°F, or Gas Mark 6 for 1 hour.

Broccoli Delight

(*Serves 4*)

1 lb (400 g) frozen broccoli florets

For the pastry crust

2 oz (50 g) oats
2 oz (50 g) wholewheat flour
1 teaspoon baking powder
1 teaspoon dried oregano
1 clove garlic, crushed
salt and pepper
2 egg whites
3 fl oz (75 ml) skimmed milk

For the topping

3 oz (75 g) low-fat Cheddar cheese, grated
3 fl oz (75 ml) skimmed milk
2 egg whites
1 small onion, finely chopped
1 clove garlic, crushed
salt and pepper to taste

Pre-heat oven at 180°C, 350°F, or Gas Mark 5. Very lightly grease or spray with non-stick cooking spray an 8 in (20 cm) baking tin.

Cook broccoli until just soft. Drain well.

To prepare the pastry crust

Put the first six pastry ingredients into a large bowl and mix well. In a separate small bowl, beat the egg whites and milk together until well blended. Add this to the dry mixture, stirring until all the ingredients are moistened. Spread this mixture evenly in the prepared baking tin.

Place the drained broccoli on top of the crust and

press down firmly with the back of a spoon so that the contents fit well into the flan case.

To prepare topping
Sprinkle the grated low-fat Cheddar cheese over the broccoli.

Combine all the remaining ingredients (milk, egg white, onion, garlic, salt and pepper) in a blender or food processor and blend until smooth. Pour this over the broccoli and cheese.

Bake uncovered for 30 minutes in the pre-heated oven. Cut into squares and serve hot.

Quick and Low-fat Courgette Lasagne

(Serves 4)

1 tablespoon olive oil
1 onion, peeled and chopped
8 oz (200 g) courgettes, diced
1 green pepper, finely diced
14 oz (350 g) tin tomatoes
2 tablespoons tomato purée
2 teaspoons bouillon powder or 1 vegetable stock cube
2 teaspoons dried basil
salt and freshly ground black pepper
8 'no pre-cook' wholemeal lasagne sheets

For the topping
½ pint (250 ml) plain natural yogurt or
low-fat fromage frais
1 egg, beaten
1 teaspoon ground cumin

Heat the oil in a frying pan and fry the onion until tender. Add the courgettes and green pepper and fry gently for a few more minutes. Add the tomatoes, tomato purée, bouillon powder (or vegetable stock cube) and dried basil, and bring the mixture to the boil. Break up the tomatoes and simmer for 10 minutes. Season well.

Place a layer of the tomato mixture on the base of a lasagne dish, cover with 4 sheets of lasagne, then repeat the tomato layer and lasagne sheets; finish with a layer of the tomato mixture.

Whisk the topping ingredients together and pour over.

Bake in a pre-heated oven at 190°C, 375°F, or Gas Mark 5 for 25–30 minutes.

Serve hot or cold with a crisp salad.

Stir-fried Vegetables with Ginger and Sesame Marinade

(Serves 4)

1½ tablespoons sunflower oil
1 onion, cut in half and shredded
12 oz (300 g) mange-tout, topped and tailed
1 large red pepper, cut into strips
10 oz (250 g) mung beansprouts
1 medium-sized Chinese cabbage, shredded

For the marinade
3 tablespoons fresh ginger juice (see below)
3 teaspoons arrowroot
3 tablespoons tamari
1 teaspoon toasted sesame oil
3 fl oz (75 ml) light stock or water

Heat the oil in a wok and quickly fry the onion

until soft. Add the mange-tout and cook for about 1 minute, stirring all the time to stop them from going brown. Add the red pepper and cook for another 3 minutes. Add the beansprouts and Chinese cabbage and cook until both look tender, stirring from time to time.

Meanwhile make the marinade by mixing all its ingredients together thoroughly.

Add the marinade to the vegetables and bring the mixture back to the boil. Cover with a lid, turn the heat down and cook for a further 3–4 minutes to finish cooking the vegetables.

Serve straight away on a bed of cooked rice.

NB The ginger juice used in this recipe can be easily made by using unpeeled root ginger. Grate the ginger and squeeze out as much of the juice as possible.

Fresh Tagliatelle with Blue Cheese Sauce

(Serves 4)

12 oz (300 g) tagliatelle

For the sauce
2 teaspoons arrowroot
½ pint (250 ml) semi-skimmed or skimmed milk
2 oz (50 g) blue cheese, crumbled
salt and freshly ground black pepper

To garnish
1–2 tablespoons fresh chopped chives

Cook the tagliatelle as indicated on the packet.
Meanwhile, place the arrowroot in a small sauce-

pan and gradually add the milk, stirring all the time. Then add the blue cheese. Bring the mixture to the boil and simmer for 2 minutes, making sure that the cheese is thoroughly melted, then season well with salt and pepper.

Serve the sauce on a bed of the tagliatelle and sprinkle the top with the chives.

Hearty Hotpot

(Serves 4)

1 onion, roughly chopped
¾ pint (375 ml) vegetable stock
6 oz (150 g) carrots, chopped
2 bay leaves
1 teaspoon caraway seeds
4 oz (100 g) swede, chopped
4 oz (100 g) parsnips, chopped
12 oz (300 g) potatoes, peeled and diced
6 oz (150 g) Brussels sprouts, halved
4 oz (100 g) tin blackeye beans, drained
4 tomatoes, peeled and chopped
3 tablespoons red wine
2 teaspoons soy sauce
salt and black pepper

In a non-stick saucepan, dry-fry the onion until soft. Add 4 fl oz (100 ml) of the vegetable stock, followed by the carrots, bay leaves and caraway seeds, and stir for a few minutes. Then add the swede, parsnips and potatoes and cook for a further 3–4 minutes. Put in the Brussels sprouts, beans, tomatoes, the remainder of the stock, the red wine and soy sauce. Place lid on pan and cook hotpot for 30 minutes or until the potatoes are soft.

Remove the bay leaves; stir the seasoning in and serve hot.

Oat and Cheese Loaf

(*Serves 4*)

8 oz (200 g) oats
1 large onion, very finely chopped
1 clove garlic, crushed
¼ teaspoon sage
¼ teaspoon thyme
¼ teaspoon ground mixed spice
salt and pepper to taste
8 oz (200 g) low-fat cottage cheese
4 egg whites

Pre-heat the oven to 180°C, 350°F, or Gas Mark 4.

Very lightly oil a 4 × 8 in (10 × 20 cm) loaf tin or spray with a non-stick cooking spray. Combine all the ingredients except the cheese and egg whites in a large bowl and mix well. In another bowl, combine the cottage cheese and egg whites and beat with a fork or wire whisk until blended. Add to the dry mixture, mixing until all the ingredients are moistened.

Press the mixture firmly into the prepared baking tin, cover with tin foil, and bake in the pre-heated oven for 25 minutes. Remove the foil and continue baking for a further 25 minutes. Allow to stand for 5 minutes before turning on to a serving plate. Serve with unlimited vegetables or salad.

Tofu Burgers

(Serves 2)

16 oz (400 g) medium tofu
2 oz (50 g) oats
½ teaspoon ground cumin
1 teaspoon chilli powder
1 clove garlic, crushed
1 onion, very finely chopped
salt and pepper to taste

Pre-heat a non-stick frying pan. Place tofu in a large bowl and mash well with a fork. Add all the other ingredients and mix well.

Shape the mixture into 6 burgers and place in the pre-heated frying pan. Cook until the burgers are brown on both sides, turning carefully.

Serve with unlimited vegetables or salad.

Tofu Indonesian-style

(Serves 4)

10 oz (250 g) packet regular tofu
1 tablespoon sunflower oil
4 oz (100 g) baby carrots, peeled and thinly sliced
6 oz (150 g) baby sweetcorn, each stick cut in half at a slant
6 oz (150 g) mange-tout, topped and tailed
4 oz (100 g) turnip or white radish, peeled and sliced
salt and freshly ground black pepper

For the sauce

2 teaspoons arrowroot
1 tablespoon tamari
1 lime leaf or bay leaf

1 small red chilli
1 small green chilli
2 in (5 cm) piece lemon grass
2 teaspoons fresh ginger juice (see note on page 258)

Cube the tofu into 20 pieces and leave it to drain on kitchen paper.

Heat the oil and sweat the vegetables in a semi-covered pan for 5 minutes, stirring from time to time.

Mix all the sauce ingredients together until smooth, add the tofu and pour the sauce and tofu over the vegetables. Replace the lid and cook for 8 minutes.

Season and serve on a bed of cooked rice.

DINNERS

Side Dishes: salads and vegetables

Carrot Salad

(See page 185)

Coleslaw

(*Serves 4*)

2 large carrots, trimmed and peeled
8 oz (200 g) white cabbage, trimmed
1 Spanish onion, peeled
4 oz (100 g) Reduced-oil Dressing (see recipe, page 280)

Wash the carrots and cabbage, then grate them and finely chop the onion. Mix together in a bowl with the Reduced-oil Dressing. Serve immediately or keep chilled and eat within 2 days.

Jacket Potatoes

1 medium-sized potato per person
salt

Scrub well even-sized potatoes and make a single cut along the top. Roll them in salt and bake in the oven at 190°C, 375°F, or Gas Mark 5 for 1½ hours (or until they give when pressed). Make cross-cuts on top of each potato and squeeze to enlarge cuts. Add filling of your choice. Serve at once.

Alternative serving suggestion
(Serves 4: Maintenance Programme)
Remove potato centres and place in a bowl, carefully preserving 'jackets'. Add 1 chopped onion, 2 oz (50 g) Shape or Tendale Cheddar-flavour cheese, coarsely grated, salt and black pepper. Mix thoroughly and replace into potato skins. Return to the oven for 10 minutes to heat through before serving.

Mashed Potatoes with Yogurt

Instead of using milk, cream or butter, mash the cooked potatoes with plain yogurt. Add a little ground pepper to make them even more delicious.

Lyonnaise Potatoes

(See page 247)

Dry-roast Potatoes

Choose medium potatoes of even size. Peel, then blanch them by putting into cold salted water and bringing to the boil.

Drain thoroughly, lightly scratch the surface of each potato with a fork, and sprinkle lightly with salt. Place in a non-stick baking tray, without fat, in a moderate oven (200°C, 400°F, Gas Mark 6) for about 1–1½ hours.

Dry-roast Parsnips

Choose even-sized medium parsnips. Peel and cut in half lengthways then blanch halved parsnips by putting into cold salted water and bringing to the boil.

Drain thoroughly and sprinkle lightly with salt. Place in a non-stick baking tray, without fat, in a moderate oven (200°C, 400°F, Gas Mark 6) for about 30 minutes. Cook until soft in the centre when pierced with a fork.

Stuffed Mushrooms

2 large mushrooms per person plus 2 or 3 extra
2 oz (50 ml) stock (vegetable or chicken)
1 teaspoon chopped onion
1 tablespoon fresh white breadcrumbs
salt and pepper
1 teaspoon parsley
pinch of dried mixed herbs

Cup mushrooms are best for this dish. Wash and

peel them and cut the stalks level with the caps as this helps prevent shrinkage.

Chop the stalks along with the extra mushrooms. Cook for 1–2 minutes in the stock with the chopped onion. Add the crumbs, seasoning, parsley and mixed herbs.

Spread this mixture on to the mushrooms and arrange them on a baking sheet or in a fireproof dish. Bake for 12–15 minutes in a moderately hot oven (200°C, 400°F, Gas Mark 6). Serve immediately.

This dish is ideal to accompany any diet dinner menu.

Garlic Mushrooms

(See pages 202–3)

Garlic Spinach

(Serves 4)

1 lb (400 g) frozen chopped spinach
1 teaspoon minced garlic
½ pint (750 ml) boiling water

Cook the spinach and garlic together for 5 minutes. Drain well, and serve.

Ratatouille

(See page 203)

DINNERS

Desserts

Fruit Sundae

(Serves 2)

8 oz (200 g) any soft fruit (blackberries, raspberries, or
strawberries – or a mixture)
6 drops liquid artificial sweetener or 1 tablespoon
granulated artificial sweetener
5 oz (125 g) plain yogurt
1 egg white

Stir the fruit, sweetener and 4 oz (100 g) of the
yogurt together thoroughly. (Save 1 oz [25 g] of
yogurt for serving).

Whisk the egg white until stiff and fold into the
fruit mixture. Spoon into serving glasses and top
with the remaining plain yogurt.

Serve immediately.

Melon Sundae

(Serves 4)

16 oz (400 g) melon fresh
10 oz (250 g) low-fat yogurt – any flavour – or low-fat
fromage frais
8 oz (200 g) green grapes

Finely chop the melon flesh and place in 4 tall
glasses. Spoon sufficient yogurt or fromage frais over
to cover the melon. Wash, halve and seed the grapes.

Divide them equally between the glasses (reserving 4 halves for decoration) and place on top. Add more yogurt or fromage frais on top and keep chilled until ready to serve. Decorate with 1 half-grape on top of each glass.

Fruit Sorbet

(Serves 6)

1 lb (400 g) fruit making ¼ pint (125 ml) fruit purée
(preferably strong-flavoured fruit, e.g. blackcurrants,
blackberries, strawberries, raspberries or black cherries;
tinned fruit may be used but remove syrup before
liquidizing
artificial sweetener to taste (if desired)
2 large egg whites

If fresh fruit is used, cook approximately 1 lb (400 g) of fruit in very little water together with a sweetening agent if desired. When the fruit is soft and the liquid well coloured, place the cooked fruit in a sieve and work the pulp with a wooden spoon until as much as possible of the fruit has passed through the mesh. Alternatively, use a liquidizer.

Allow to cool and place the purée in a metal or plastic container, cover with a lid and freeze until it begins to set. When a layer of purée approximately ½ in (1 cm) thick has frozen, remove the mixture from the freezer and stir it so that the mixture is a soft crystallized consistency.

Whisk the two egg whites until stiff and standing in peaks. Fold into the semi-frozen purée to give a marbled effect. Immediately return the mixture to the freezer and freeze until firm.

Serve straight from the freezer.

Pineapple and Orange Sorbet

(Serves 6)

small tin crushed pineapple in natural juice
1 orange, peeled and chopped
liquid sweetener
8 fl oz (200 ml) fresh orange juice
2 egg whites

Crush pineapple well and mix with chopped orange, and orange juice. Sweeten to taste. Place in a plastic container in your freezer or the freezer compartment in your refrigerator. Freeze until half frozen.

Whisk egg whites until stiff. Turn out half-frozen mixture into a mixing bowl and fold in whisked egg whites.

Return mixture to freezer until firm.

Fruit Jelly with Fromage Frais

(Serves 4)

1 pint (500 ml) white grape juice or apple juice
½ oz (12.5 g) gelatine
4 oz (100 g) fromage frais

Heat the fruit juice through, at the same time adding the gelatine and stirring until it dissolves. Pour into individual dishes. Leave to set in the refrigerator.

Serve with fromage frais.

Apple Jelly with Fromage Frais

(Serves 4)

stewed apple (made with artificial sweetener to taste)
1 packet jelly

2 cups water
4 oz (100 g) fromage frais

Make up the stewed apple and leave to cool. Spoon the apple into individual dishes.

Make up the jelly with the 2 cups of water and then pour it over the apple in the individual dishes. Leave to set.

When ready to serve, top with fromage frais.

Summer Delight

(See pages 181–2)

Apple and Blackcurrant Whip

(*Serves 4*)

1 lb (400 g) cooking apples
2 fl oz (50 ml) water
saccharin or liquid sweetener to taste
2 egg whites
2 tablespoons low-calorie blackcurrant jam or 4 oz (100 g) fresh or frozen blackcurrants

Peel, core and slice apples and cook with the water until they become a thick pulp. Add sweetener. Set aside to cool.

Whisk egg whites until stiff and fold gently into cooled apple purée.

Pile into individual sundae dishes or a medium-sized serving dish. Swirl jam or blackcurrant fruit on the top to give a marble/ripple effect.

Raspberry Mousse

(Serves 4)

8 oz (200 g) fresh or frozen raspberries *or* 7 oz (175 g)
tin raspberries in natural juice
4 oz (100 g) natural apple juice
liquid sweetener, approx. 15 drops
1 teaspoon gelatine
2 egg whites
4 teaspoons raspberry yogurt
12 fresh raspberries to decorate

Place raspberries and apple juice in a liquidizer and blend until smooth. Strain through a sieve into a basin. Add liquid sweetener to taste.

Dissolve gelatine in 3 teaspoons of water in a cup over very hot water. Add to raspberry purée and stir well.

Whisk egg whites until they form peaks. Fold into purée.

Pour mixture into four tall sundae glasses or a serving dish. Decorate with raspberry yogurt and fresh raspberries just before serving.

Pears in Red Wine

(Serves 4)

6 ripe pears, peeled but left whole
2 wineglasses red wine
2 fl oz (50 ml) water
2 oz (50 g) brown sugar
½ level teaspoon cinnamon or ground ginger

To microwave

Combine wine, water, sugar and spice in a glass jug and microwave on *high* for approximately 4 minutes or until boiling.

Place the pears in a deep soufflé dish, pour wine sauce over them and cover with cling film. Microwave on *high* for approximately 5 minutes or until just tender but retaining their shape.

To cook on stove

Combine wine, water, sugar and spice in a large saucepan, and bring to the boil. Add the pears to the pan and simmer for 10–15 minutes, turning the pears carefully from time to time to ensure even colouring.

Serve hot or cold. Maintenance dieters may serve with low-fat, low-calorie ice cream.

Pears in Meringue

(*Serves 6*)

6 ripe dessert pears, peeled but left whole
10 fl oz (250 ml) apple juice
3 egg whites
6 oz (150 g) caster sugar

Cook the pears in the apple juice until just tender. Cut a slice off the bottom of each pear to enable them to sit in a dish without falling over. Place them, well spaced out, in an ovenproof dish.

Put the egg whites in a large and completely grease-free bowl and whisk them, preferably with a balloon whisk or rotary beater as these make more volume than an electric whisk.

When the egg whites are firm and stand in peaks, whisk into them 1 tablespoon of the caster sugar for 1 minute. Fold the remainder of the sugar in with a metal spoon, cutting the egg whites rather than mixing them.

Place the egg white and sugar mixture into a large piping bag equipped with a metal nozzle (any pattern) and pipe a pyramid around each pear, starting from the base and working upwards. Place in a moderate oven (160°C, 325°F, Gas Mark 3), and cook until firm and golden.

Serve hot or cold. Maintenance dieters may serve with low-fat, low-calorie ice cream if desired.

Pineapple in Kirsch

(Serves 4)

1 fresh pineapple
1 liqueur/sherry glass Kirsch

Remove skin and core from the pineapple and slice the flesh into rings.

Sprinkle the Kirsch over the fruit and place in a refrigerator for at least 12 hours to marinate. Keep turning the fruit to ensure even flavouring.

Maintenance dieters may serve with low-fat, low-calorie ice cream if desired.

Oranges Grand Marnier and Yogurt Sauce

(Serves 4)

1 wineglass medium to sweet white wine *or* fresh orange juice

1 sherry glass Grand Marnier liqueur
1 tablespoon demerara sugar, or liquid artificial
sweetener if preferred
6 oranges

For the sauce
8 oz (200 g) low-fat natural yogurt
2 tablespoons Grand Marnier

Heat the white wine (or orange juice) with the liqueur in a saucepan. Add the sugar, bring to the boil and simmer until the sugar is dissolved. Allow to cool. Add liquid artificial sweetener if desired.

Carefully peel the oranges with a very sharp knife to remove all pith. This can be done by slicing across the top of the orange and then using this flat end as a base. Cut strips of peel away from the top downwards so that the orange is completely free from the white membranes of the pith. Squeeze the peel to extract any juice and pour this into the wine mixture.

Cut the oranges across to give round slices of equal size and place in the cool liquid. Allow to stand in a refrigerator for at least 12 hours.

Just before serving, mix the yogurt with the Grand Marnier and serve this sauce separately.

Gooseberry Surprise

(Serves 4)

1 lb (400 g) gooseberries, topped and tailed
4 tablespoons water
1 teaspoon lemon juice
10 artificial sweetener tablets
4 tablespoons semolina
1 pint (500 ml) skimmed milk (in addition to allowance)

273

green food colouring
5 oz (125 g) natural yogurt

Reserve 4 gooseberries for decoration and place the remainder in a pan with the water and the lemon juice. Cook on a low heat until soft. Near the end of cooking add the artificial sweetener tablets, or liquid sweetener if you prefer. When the fruit is thoroughly cooked, pass the pulp through a sieve in order to remove the pips and hard skin.

Mix the semolina with a little of the skimmed milk in a bowl and bring the remaining milk to boiling point. Gradually pour the hot milk into the semolina, stirring all the time. Return to the pan and boil for 3 minutes, stirring continuously.

Remove from the heat and add the gooseberry purée and colouring. Divide into four individual dishes, allow to cool and place in the refrigerator. Just before serving, top with natural yogurt and decorate with the reserved gooseberries.

Peach Brûlée

(*Serves 1*)

3 oz (75 g) tin peaches in natural juice
3 oz (75 g) low-fat yogurt or fromage frais
1 tablespoon demerara sugar

Switch on the grill at *high* setting.

Drain the peaches and place in a ramekin dish. Spoon the yogurt or fromage frais over the fruit, flatten the surface and sprinkle the demerara sugar evenly on top. Immediately place under the pre-heated hot grill, and watch it all the time until the sugar caramelizes.

Serve immediately.

Hot Cherries

(Serves 4)

15 oz (375 g) tin black cherries
3 fl oz (75 ml) cherry brandy (optional)
2 teaspoons arrowroot
4 oz (100 g) ice cream (non-Cornish variety)

Strain the cherries reserving the juice. Heat the cherry juice in a pan, add cherry brandy if desired, and thicken with enough slaked arrowroot (approximately 2 teaspoons mixed with water) to make a syrup. Stir the cherries in and pour this over 1 oz (25 g) low-fat, low-calorie ice cream per person.

Serve immediately.

Kim's Cake

(1 serving = ½ in [1.25 cm] slice)

1 lb (400 g) dried mixed fruit
1 mug hot black tea (or alternative [see below])
1 mug soft brown sugar
2 mugs self-raising flour
1 beaten egg

Soak the dried fruit – for a birthday-type fruit cake, add some cherries – overnight in the hot black tea.

As an alternative, use a fruit infusion herbal tea instead of black tea. This gives a delicious smell and flavour to the cake. A raspberry or strawberry flavour is particularly recommended.

The next day, mix all ingredients (including the tea) together, then place into a 2 lb (800 g) loaf tin or round cake tin. Bake for 2 hours at 160°C, 325°F, or Gas Mark 3. Serve hot or cold. (This cake can be frozen.)

Banana and Sultana Cake

(1 serving = ½ in [1.3 cm] slice)

1 lb 3 oz (475 g) ripe bananas (5 large peeled)
2 eggs, beaten
6 oz (150 g) brown sugar
4 oz (100 g) sultanas
8 oz (200 g) self-raising flour

Mash bananas; add eggs, sugar and sultanas and then mix the flour in. Place in a lined 2 lb (800 g) loaf tin or cake tin.

Bake for 1¼ hours in a pre-heated oven at 180°C, 350°F, or Gas Mark 4. Store in an airtight tin for 24 hours before serving. Suitable for freezing.

This can be an economical recipe as very ripe bananas can often be purchased cheaply. Because of the number of portions that can be served from this loaf, the egg content need not be included in your allowance of 2 eggs per week.

Sultana Cake

(Serves 6)

1½ cups self-raising wholemeal flour (fine stoneground)
¾ cup Branflakes
1½ cups sultanas
1½ cups skimmed milk

Mix flour and Branflakes together in a bowl, add the sultanas and mix well. Pour the milk into the mixture and stir well.

Bake in a non-stick muffin pan at 200°C, 400°F, or Gas Mark 6 for 5–8 minutes until cooked.

To serve, spread with a little apricot jam.

Apple Gâteau

(Serves 8: Maintenance dieters only)

Makes one 8 in (20 cm) cake.

For the cake

3 eggs
4½ oz (112 g) caster sugar
3 oz (75 g) plain flour, sifted
pinch of salt

For the filling

1 lb (400 g) eating apples, peeled, cored and sliced
grated rind and juice of 1 lemon
1 tablespoon apricot jam
artificial sweetener for apples if desired
1 teaspoon icing sugar

For the cake: Very lightly grease an 8 in (20 cm) cake

277

tin. Dust with caster sugar, then with flour. Shake out the excess.

Place the eggs and caster sugar in a mixing bowl and whisk with an electric whisk/mixer for 5 minutes at top speed. When thick and mousse-like, fold in the sifted flour and salt.

Pour into the prepared tin. Bake in the centre of a moderately hot oven (190°C, 375°F, Gas Mark 5) for 25 minutes or until golden brown and shrunk from the edges of the tin a little. Run a blunt knife around the inside of the tin and turn out the cake on to a wire rack to cool.

For the filling: Place the apple slices in a pan with the grated rind and juice of a lemon and the jam. Heat slowly. Add the artificial sweetener to taste if required. Cover and cook until the apples are just tender.

When the cake is cool, slice it across with a large knife to make two layers. Spread the bottom half with the cooled apple filling and cover with the top half of the cake. Sprinkle with icing sugar on top.

Diet Rice Pudding

(*Serves 4*)

1 pint (500 ml) low-fat skimmed milk
1 oz (25 g) pudding rice
approx. 20 saccharin tablets or 20 drops liquid sweetener
pinch of nutmeg (optional)

Place all ingredients except nutmeg in an ovenproof dish. Sprinkle the nutmeg over the top. Cook in the oven for 2–2½ hours at 150°C, 300°F, or Gas Mark 2. If the pudding is still sloppy 30–40 minutes before it is to be eaten, raise the oven temperature to 160°C, 325°F, or Gas Mark 3.

Serve hot or cold. If you intend to serve cold, remove from oven while still very moist as it will become stiffer and drier when cool.

Baked Stuffed Apple

(Serves 1)

1 large cooking apple
1 oz (25 g) dried fruit
1 teaspoon honey
2 tablespoons natural low-fat yogurt

Remove the core from the apple but leave the apple intact. Score with a sharp knife around the 'waist' of the apple, cutting through only the skin. Mix together the dried fruit and the honey and pile into the centre of the apple where the core has been removed.

Place in an ovenproof dish and bake in a moderate oven (200°C, 400°F, or Gas Mark 6) for about 30 minutes, or until cooked.

Serve with the yogurt poured over the top.

Low-fat Custard

(See pages 284–5)

DRESSING AND SAUCES

Oil-free Vinaigrette Dressing

3 tablespoons white wine vinegar or cider vinegar
1 tablespoon lemon juice
½ teaspoon black pepper
½ teaspoon salt
1 teaspoon sugar
½ teaspoon French mustard
chopped herbs (thyme, marjoram, basil or parsley)

Place all the ingredients in a container, seal, then shake well. Taste and add more salt or sugar as desired.

Oil-free Orange and Lemon Vinaigrette

4 oz (100 g) wine vinegar
4 tablespoons lemon juice
4 tablespoons orange juice
grated rind of 1 lemon
½ teaspoon French mustard
1 pinch of garlic salt
freshly ground black pepper

Place all the ingredients in a bowl and mix thoroughly. Keep in a refrigerator and use this dressing within two days.

Reduced-oil Dressing

Mix 3 tablespoons reduced-oil salad dressing (e.g. Waistline or Weight Watchers) with 5 oz (125 g) plain low-fat yogurt. Add salt and pepper.

Keep in a refrigerator for up to 2 days.

Yogurt Dressing

5 oz (125 g) natural yogurt
good squeeze of lemon juice
salt and freshly ground black pepper

Mix all the ingredients together and serve as a dressing for salad.

Yogurt and Mint Dressing

5 oz (125 g) natural yogurt
1 teaspoon mint sauce
salt and freshly ground black pepper

Mix all the ingredients together and keep refrigerated. Chill before using and serve on salads, jacket potatoes, etc.

Garlic or Mint Yogurt Dip

(See pages 198–9)

Seafood Dressing (1)

(*Serves 2*)

2 tablespoons tomato ketchup
1 tablespoon reduced-oil salad dressing (e.g. Waistline)
squeeze of lemon juice

Mix all ingredients together and use as allowed.

Seafood Dressing (2)

(Serves 2)

1 tablespoons tomato ketchup
1 tablespoon reduced-oil salad dressing (e.g. Waistline)
4 tablespoons natural yogurt
dash of Tabasco sauce
salt and pepper to taste

Mix all the ingredients together and store in a refrigerator. Serve within 2 days.

Barbecue Sauce

(Serves 2)

1 teaspoon plain flour
⅓ pint (167 ml) potato stock
1 tablespoon soy sauce
dash Worcestershire sauce
salt and pepper
4 oz (100 g) tin tomatoes

Skim off all fat from grill pan after cooking meat or poultry, leaving any sediment. To this fat-free sediment add the flour and a tablespoon of the stock. Stir well and cook very gently for 2–3 minutes.

Draw aside and blend in potato stock, sauces and seasonings. Return to heat and stir until boiling. Add the tinned tomatoes, which should be finely chopped (scissor snipped). Simmer for a minute or until it takes on a creamy consistency.

This sauce goes well with kebabs and grilled or baked chicken.

Garlic Sauce

8 oz (200 g) tin tomatoes
3 cloves garlic, peeled and finely chopped
1 teaspoon dried oregano or basil
salt and freshly ground black pepper

Place all the ingredients in a saucepan and simmer gently until piping hot. Serve as a sauce with steak or chicken.

White Sauce

½ pint (250 ml) skimmed milk
1 onion, peeled and sliced
6 peppercorns
1 bay leaf
salt and freshly ground black pepper
1 dessertspoon cornflour

Heat all but 2 fl oz (50 ml) of the milk in a non-stick saucepan, adding the onion, peppercorns, bay leaf and seasoning. Cover the pan and simmer for 5 minutes. Turn off heat and leave milk mixture to stand, with the lid on, for a further 30 minutes or until it is time to thicken and serve the sauce.

Mix remaining milk with cornflour and, when almost time to serve, strain the infused milk, add the cornflour mixture and reheat slowly, stirring continuously, until it comes to the boil. If it begins to thicken too quickly, remove from heat and stir very fast to mix well. Cook for 3–4 minutes and serve immediately.

Parsley Sauce

As White Sauce, but add chopped fresh parsley or dried parsley to taste during final cooking.

Gravy

If you are roasting a joint, you can make 'low-fat' gravy using the meat juices by following the procedure below.

Bake the joint on a rack in the oven. Drain and discard the fat from the roasting tin, retaining the meat juices, and add 2–3 cups of water to the tin. Heat to boiling point, at the same time scraping the brown residue off the bottom of the roasting tin and stirring it to mix with the water and meat juices.

Pour the liquid into a bowl and leave to cool. Place in the refrigerator to stand overnight. Remove from the refrigerator the next day and scrape off any fat lying on the top of the liquid. You can either freeze the liquid to use for gravy later or else place it in a saucepan, heat and thicken with a little cornflour mixed with water, to serve immediately.

Low-fat Custard

(*Serves 2*)

½ pint (250 ml) skimmed milk
1 tablespoon custard powder
8 saccharin tablets or 15 drops liquid sweetener

Heat most of the milk in a non-stick saucepan. Mix the remainder of the milk with the custard powder

and add slowly to the heated milk, stirring continuously.

Add saccharin tablets and continue to stir until
boiling. Simmer for approximately 5 minutes.

DRINKS

St Clements

slimline orange
slimline bitter lemon

Pour half a bottle of each into a tall glass filled with
ice. Top up as required.

For an extra-special drink use freshly squeezed
orange juice with the bitter lemon.

Orange/Lemon Barley Drink

3 large or 4 small oranges or lemons
4 pints (2 litres) water
4 oz (100 g) pearl barley (optional)
16 oz (400 g) jar Nutrasweet or Canderel
2 oz (50 g) citric acid

Peel off zest of fruit with a potato peeler and remove
pith. Boil the peel in 2 pints (1 litre) of the water
for 20–30 minutes. Strain, reserving the liquid.

Place the pearl barley in the other 2 pints (1 litre)
of water, bring to the boil, then simmer for 1 hour.
Strain, reserving the liquid.

Combine the two reserved liquids and add the
Nutrasweet or Canderel and citric acid. Add juice

of lemons/oranges when liquid mixture is cool in order not to destroy the Vitamin C.

Grapefruit Fizz

unsweetened grapefruit juice
slimline tonic water

Pour approximately 4 fl oz (100 ml) unsweetened grapefruit juice into a tall glass and add plenty of ice. Add the slimline tonic and continue topping up with the remainder of the tonic.

This drink is an excellent 'filler' before a meal.

Ginger Orange

5 fl oz (125 ml) unsweetened orange juice
5 fl oz (125 ml) slimline ginger ale

Mix in a tall glass filled with ice.

Garnish with sliced orange, lemon and mint leaves.

Pacific Delight

Mix 2 fl oz (50 ml) lime cordial with slimline ginger ale in a tall glass filled with ice.

Caribbean Surprise

5 fl oz (125 ml) unsweetened pineapple juice
slimline ginger ale

Mix in a tall glass filled with ice. Top up with ginger ale as desired.

Garnish with a cherry, pineapple, orange slice and pineapple or mint leaves on a cocktail stick.

Sludge Gulper

4 fl oz (100 ml) unsweetened orange juice
1 can diet cola

Pour orange juice into a tall glass filled with ice. Pour on the diet cola.

Serve with a straw.

Apple Cola

Mix a can of diet cola with one can of Appletize. Serve in tall glasses with ice.

Pineapple Sludge

5 fl oz (125 ml) pineapple juice
1 can diet cola

Half fill a glass with ice, pour the pineapple juice over and top up with diet cola. Although the appearance of the drink may be off-putting, the taste is delicious!

Spritzer

5 fl oz (125 ml) white wine
sparkling mineral water or soda water

Pour the wine into a large-sized wineglass and add the mineral or soda water. This provides a long and very enjoyable drink that can accompany a meal or just be drunk for pleasure socially.

Buck's Fizz

(This drink is recommended to celebrate rediscovering your youthful figure)

1 bottle champagne, well chilled
freshly squeezed orange juice, well chilled

Fill champagne flutes one-third full with orange juice. Fill to the top with champagne.

Cheers!

10
The value of exercise

I think we have established that my Hip and Thigh Diet really does slim hips and thighs very effectively indeed. But can we do any *more* to improve the contours of our trimmed down body?

Regular exercise, as well as making us fitter, can help to reduce cellulite and increase muscle tone, giving us a better body shape. But there's one thing we need to establish firmly before we go any further. It is impossible to turn fat into muscle just as it is impossible to turn a cat into a dog. Not only are fat and muscle made from completely different compositions, they also fulfil different functions. If you have got an excess amount of fat across your tummy or on your thighs, the most effective exercises in the world will not get rid of it. However, exercise does enable us to increase our metabolic rate and also to burn away fat, so by asking our body to use more energy than we are taking in in the form of food we *can* help burn away the excesses and reap the rewards of a trimmer body.

As part of your preparation for your campaign towards a leaner, fitter and healthier body, it is wise to prepare yourself for increased physical activity.

Muscles that have not been exercised for years will prove very painful if overworked when you first start to exercise them again – and pain is likely to discourage you from any further attempts! We tell ourselves that it is too late, that the damage and abuse we have caused ourselves over the years is irreparable. Of course this is not in fact true. No matter how unfit or unused to physical activity we are, we can change our fitness level surprisingly swiftly if we exercise regularly. Everyone should start slowly, and gradually build up their level of activity. Perhaps the most crucial factor is finding a form of exercise you actually enjoy. Exercising to music is my particular favourite and I also try to work out in our gym twice a week.

When my first Hip and Thigh Diet proved so successful some of the ladies at my exercise classes said, 'Oh, you won't have time to take our classes soon – you'll be too busy doing more exciting things.' They couldn't be more wrong. I love taking my classes and I love my ladies – a cheerful and friendly crowd if ever there was one! Not only do I enjoy seeing them each week, but actually doing the exercises to pop music in the luxurious surroundings of the Holiday Inn is totally pleasurable. I love it. And that's it – we should *all* aim for enjoyment, not punishment.

My husband Mike plays squash and golf regularly, as well as working out in the gym, and my daughter Dawn attends my weekly exercise class and swims as often as possible. She also exercises to videos at home. Exercising shouldn't be a chore; but ought to become a normal part of our lifestyle. The benefits of regular exercise are obvious: improved fitness, a healthier heart, a toned and more attractive body shape and a higher metabolic rate. At the same

time, exercise burns up extra calories . . . so what
are we waiting for?

Eileen Forrest wrote:

'Five years ago my husband and I bought our
own business, a post office and newsagents shop.
I then weighed 9½ st (60.3 kg) and very soon the
weight began to pile on. My temptation to try all
the sweets got the better of me. How silly I was,
but at the time I didn't notice all the weight going
on. Before I knew it I went to a staggering 11 st
2 lbs (70.7 kg) and just felt awful. I went to the
doctor because I was feeling very tired and that is
when I discovered my weight gain. I was so
depressed. He put me on a diet and I lost a stone
(6.4 kg) in a month, but somehow I just could not
stick to it and the weight went on again. Then, two
years ago, I bought your *Hip and Thigh Diet* book.
I stuck to the diet religiously and went down to 9 st
2 lbs (58 kg). My weight kept steady, but I still
felt I could lose a bit more to feel good.

Just after Christmas last year I bought your
Whole Body Programme tape. That was the real
turning point for me. I am absolutely hooked on
the exercises. I exercise at least six times a week
and feel like a new woman.

I am forty-two years of age, 5 ft 2 ins (1.58 m)
tall and now weigh a nimble 8 st 11 lbs (51.3 kg).
I have lost 4 ins (10 cm) from my thighs, 4 ins
(10 cm) from my waist and 4½ ins (11 cm) from
my hips. I have gone from a size 14 to a size 10. I
cannot thank you enough. Your diet is a way of
life for me now. It has given me more self-

confidence and above all my husband says I look great.'

As soon as you have read this section, think carefully about how you can increase your physical activity over the next week. The next chapter illustrates a variety of exercises which are specifically designed to improve the contour of your hips and thighs. They have been developed over a period of years and I believe these are the ultimate in effective exercises for this area. (In 1992 I brought out a further video on this same subject. This video is part of my *Top to Toe Collection*, published by the BBC and available from all video outlets.)

If we combine specific body-toning exercises with general aerobic activity such as brisk walking, swimming, jogging, cycling etc., we are doing all we possibly can to improve the shape and physical condition of our body. Activities that can be enjoyed by the whole family are a particularly good idea as not only can we encourage each other but we also ensure that we practise regularly. Working out with a friend or your family acts as an insurance in not letting the activity slip.

Aim to do something physical each day. Exercise should be energetic enough to make you puff, but not cause you to be so out of breath that you can't talk normally. Keep a record of your activity and the duration, repetitions and intensity. Make a note of how you felt afterwards. If you repeat the same activity the next day, aim to increase the intensity or the duration. If you can't exercise every day, try to do something at least three times a week.

There are five elements contributing to physical fitness. These are: Stamina, Muscular endurance, Strength, Flexibility and Motor fitness.

Stamina

This is built up through sustained aerobic exercise when the body is working hard enough to achieve a heart rate of between 60 per cent and 85 per cent of its maximum. Our maximum heart rate per minute can be calculated by deducting our age from 220. Aerobic exercise includes: jogging, swimming, step classes, aerobics and sports such as tennis. Moderate stamina exercises are often used within a warming-up programme of exercises.

Muscular endurance

This is developed by training a group of muscles to overcome resistance over a period of time. The source of the resistance can be gravity or your own body weight, or you can use a rubber band, ball or light external weights. As we become fitter we can increase the muscular endurance by increasing the number of repetitions of each exercise. It is these exercises that are particularly important when we are aiming to improve the shape of our hips and thighs.

Strength

Exercises to develop strength can incorporate the use of external weights or we can use our own body weight and gravity to give the necessary resistance. To become *stronger*, we need to increase the resistance and not the number of repetitions. Strength exercises are used to build muscle.

Flexibility

Developing flexibility or suppleness involves length-
ening the muscles by using a wider range of movements, particularly stretching exercises. As we
become more supple we are able to stretch the
muscles further. Flexibility enables us to have a
better posture, to carry ourselves well.

Motor fitness

The relationship between the brain and the muscle
action determines our level of motor fitness as it
relates to co-ordination, balance and the reaction
time taken in the performance of different movements. Dancers have a high level of motor fitness
and this is something we can all develop over a
period of time. In a class situation, someone with a
high motor fitness level will achieve greater benefit
because the quality of his/her movements will be
improved since he/she is able to follow closely the
movements of the teacher.

Ten essential tips for exercising

1. Always check with your doctor before starting
this or any other kind of exercise and diet programme. If during the exercises you feel any pain or
discomfort, stop immediately. If you feel one particular exercise doesn't suit you because it is uncomfortable to do, leave it out.

2. Movements should always be rhythmic, controlled and slow – never jerky or hurried, which
would eliminate the benefits.

3. ALWAYS warm up before any form of exercise.

4. Never overwork or overstretch your body. Look

for warning signals such as feeling faint, pain, nausea and so on.

5. Relate the level of your workout to your environment (e.g. type of flooring, fresh air, heat, etc.) and your own physical condition. If you haven't exercised for 30 years, take it very slowly at the start and increase your activity as you become fitter.

6. Always wear suitable clothing for exercise. Correct footwear is particularly important, especially for aerobic exercise.

7. If you become fit enough to do many repetitions of some of the exercises included in this programme, beware of possible overuse of some of your joints. To remedy this, go on to the next exercise that uses different muscles and joints, then return to the original exercise. Vary the high-impact and low-impact aerobic exercises in the same way.

8. You should be able to feel the muscle that is 'working' in the strength and endurance exercises. If you can't, check that you are doing the exercise correctly by carefully re-reading the instructions. Do the same with the stretching exercises. If you can't feel the muscle being stretched, double check your position with that in the picture.

9. Plan a time to do your exercises each day and try to stick to it. Be disciplined about your workout. This is your opportunity to have a great new body in just a few weeks. Work out with a friend or partner for greater enjoyment. The exercises are suitable for men and women.

10. Never exercise immediately after a meal. Wait at least 1 to 1½ hours.

11
The Hip and Thigh Workout

These exercises will significantly improve your body shape if practised regularly. Do not rush them, but try and set aside a particular time of the day, and play some of your favourite pop music to help you improve the momentum of the movements. The amount and the regularity of your workout will be determined by how badly you want to be in good shape! Another very important point is that when we exercise, more oxygen reaches our skin. This is particularly valuable for anyone on a weight-reducing diet as it enables the skin to shrink as the pounds disappear, leaving the body in a firm and toned condition without any flabby skin.

Here are a couple of letters from dieters who wrote to me to this effect.

Marina Escott wrote:

'I thought you would be interested to know that I have had a weight problem all my life; in my younger years I was actually 17 st 3 lbs (109.3 kg) a fact I feel ashamed to admit. To cut a very long story short, I dieted, joined clubs and lost around 2 to 3 stones (12.7–19 kg) only to pile the pounds back on as soon as I stopped dieting.

As you can imagine the loose ugly skin at the tops of my legs and especially around my middle caused me much distress to say the least. My hubby and daughter often said I would never get rid of the loose skin unless I had an operation. Well, Rosemary, I am thrilled to tell you that it has gone! My family can't believe their eyes. It's entirely due to the exercises in your *Whole Body Programme* video which I practise nearly every day, including weekends and holidays. I even take an audio cassette of the exercises when we go away to our caravan, so I can still practise them to music. I take my mat and do the exercises on the patio (outside the caravan) with neighbours and anyone else looking on and pulling my leg, but to no avail. I just shout, 'come and join me'.

People say how slim I look and it's all thanks to your sensible low-fat eating plan and exercises. Believe me, to actually see all my unsightly skin disappearing before my very eyes is enough to make me continue with the exercises.

I benefit from feeling so well. I tell all my friends I feel better now at fifty-six years of age than I did when I was thirty. My husband agrees wholeheartedly and says I look better too!'

Margaret Ainsworth wrote:

'Thank you very much for your Hip and Thigh Diet. I have gone from 13½ stone (85.7 kg) to 11 stone (69.8 kg). My measurements were 43–36–45 ins (107–90–112 cm) and 47 ins (117 cm) widest part, to 38–28–39 ins (95–70–97 cm) and 41 ins (102 cm) widest part. I have lost 3½ ins (8.7 cm) off each thigh, 3½ ins

(8.7 cm) from each knee and 2 ins (5 cm) from each upper arm. I had a weight problem all my life (I am forty-two years old) and tried numerous diets with poor results. But now I get compliments every day on how fantastic I look! I can now get into jeans. I wear size 14 when I used to wear size 20. I also get compliments on how wonderful my skin and my hair look. I haven't always been able to strictly follow the diet, since in my job I often have to eat food prepared for me, with inadequate choice to fit in with the diet, but I have kept to the diet as closely as possible. The main thing is that it has been easy to stick to and I haven't had any urges to binge and blow it all, as in the past.

I intend to continue and get down to 9 stone (57 kg) which I think will be about right for me – I'm about 5 ft 5 ins (1.65 m) tall. I should also mention that I followed your exercise programme which has helped tremendously too.

I've been told I look twenty years younger and have been mistaken for my fourteen-year-old daughter's sister! This makes so much difference to me and I'm sure to many others like me.'

Exercise is the key to enabling the skin to return to a firm and taut texture. If you have a significant amount of weight to lose, in addition to following the diet, it is absolutely imperative to exercise to enable the skin to shrink and firm up. Not only will it make your skin look better, but it will also make you *feel* better. Fitness can be achieved by almost everyone, so let's go and enjoy it!

The warm-up

Warming-up our body with gentle exercises prepares the body and mind for exercise, enabling us to maximize our performance both physically and mentally. Warming-up exercises prepare the heart and lungs for the additional work they will have to do; help to prevent soreness and injury in the major muscle groups; and rehearse the movements of the exercises that will follow, thus enhancing our performance. Exercises performed correctly are obviously more effective.

There are three elements of a warm-up:

1. Mobilizing. When we take our joints gently through a range of movements the body prepares them for action in various ways, including secreting synovial fluid which allows the joint actions to be smoother, easier and safer.
2. Pulse raising. By practising a few exercises that use the large muscle groups we increase our heart rate and prepare our cardiovascular system for exercise.
3. Preparatory stretches. We need to stretch our muscles to reduce the chance of injury. Muscles are like elastic and become more pliable when warm. Warming and stretching them prevents injury and improves performance.

Warm-up I: mobilizer

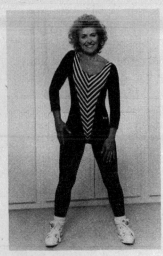

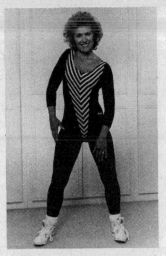

1 Shoulder raises
Standing with your feet slightly apart and your knees slightly bent, raise and lower one shoulder 8 times. Repeat with the other shoulder.

2 Shoulder rotation (single)
Rotate one shoulder backwards 8 times. Repeat with the other shoulder. Then rotate one shoulder forwards 8 times and repeat with the other shoulder.

Warm-up I: mobilizer

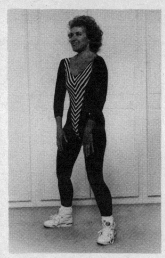

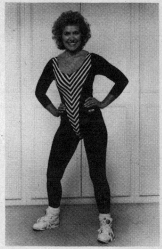

3 Shoulder rotation (doubles)
Rotate both shoulders backwards
8 times, then forwards 8 times.
Repeat sequence 8 times in each
direction.

4 Pelvic rotation
With hands on hips, rotate your
hips 4 times in a clockwise
direction and then 4 times in an
anti-clockwise direction. Repeat
in both directions for 4 rotations
each way.

Warm-up I: mobilizer

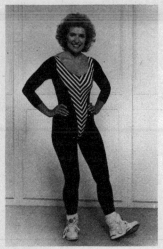
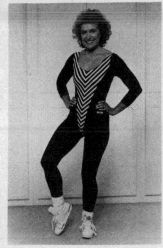

5 Heel and toe tapping
With hands on hips, tap the heel of one foot and then the toe. Repeat 8 times (8 heels and 8 toes) and then repeat with the other foot.

6 Arm swinging, kicking across
Swinging your arms gently from side to side, kick alternate legs across your body. Repeat with alternate legs 16 times (8 kicks with each leg).

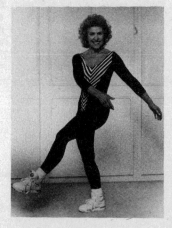

Warm-up II: pulse raiser

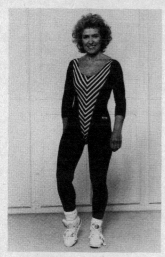

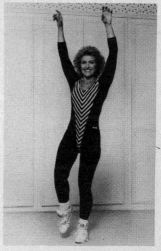

7 Walking jog
Do a walking jog on the spot for 30 steps (15 with each foot). Swing your arms as you step.

8 Marching, arm raising
Marching on the spot with big leg movements, raise your arms out to the sides and up above your head and then down as you place each foot back on the floor. Repeat 20 times (10 for each foot).

Warm-up II: pulse raiser

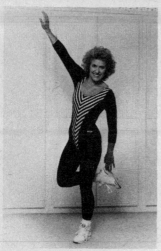

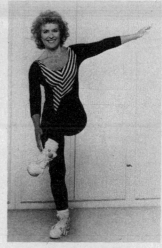

9 Kick and touch
Kick your right leg behind the left one and try to touch the foot with your left hand; at the same time allow your right hand to swing upwards. Repeat to the other side. Repeat this sequence 20 times (10 for each leg).

10 Alternate foot raises
Raise one foot towards the opposite hand then repeat with the other foot. Repeat 16 times (8 with each foot).

Warm-up II: pulse raiser

11 Marching, arms out and in
Marching on the spot with large
steps, take your arms out to the
sides then into the centre. Repeat
24 times (12 with each leg).

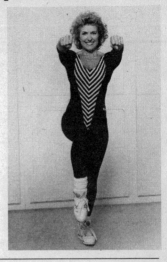

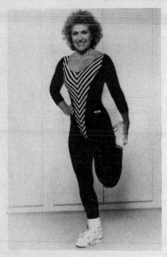

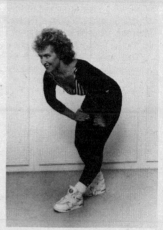

12 Front thigh stretch
Standing with your feet together, bend your left leg and take hold of its foot with your left hand. Stretch the front thigh muscles by easing your foot as close to your seat as possible. Do not strain. Hold the position for 6 seconds before slowly releasing the leg to the floor. Bend the other leg, hold it with your other hand and stretch the muscles as before, holding the position for 6 seconds. Release your leg slowly to the floor.

13 Hamstring stretch
Stand with one foot behind the other and with your feet hip-width apart, feet pointing straight ahead. Keep the front leg straight and bend the back leg, lowering your hips without straining. Place your hands on your thighs (not on your knees) and hold for 8 seconds. Proceed to the next exercise.

Warm-up III: preparatory stretches

14 Calf stretch
Maintaining the position of the
Hamstring stretch, raise the toes
of your front foot, keeping your
front leg straight and your heel
on the floor. Hold for a count of
8. This stretches the calf. Relax
and then repeat Exercises 13 and
14 with the other leg forward.

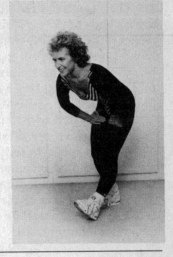

Aerobic Workout

Aerobic exercise strengthens our heart and also burns body fat. It improves the capacity and efficiency of the cardiorespiratory system so that it delivers more oxygen to the working muscles. It improves muscular endurance, lowers our blood fat levels and helps to lower blood pressure. There are also various other benefits in the reduction of risk factors associated with coronary heart disease.

The energy source of aerobic exercise is oxygen. We breathe more heavily during aerobic exercise because the body demands a greater supply of oxygen. Providing the oxygen supply is maintained, aerobic exercise can be continued for a long time (as in the case of a marathon runner). Aerobic exercise involves the larger muscle groups (those of the arms and legs) and can be high-impact or low-impact, high-intensity or low-intensity. High-impact aerobic exercises involve both feet leaving the ground (e.g. jumping, jogging or skipping) whereas low-impact exercise is when one foot always remains on the floor (e.g. a walking jog, knee raises or marching). The intensity level is determined by the size and speed of a movement. Someone who finds it difficult to do high-impact aerobics can still work out very energetically if large and high arm movements are included.

The aerobic exercises recommended here can be adapted to your individual capability. If you do not wish to perform high-impact movements, keep the exercises low-impact by eliminating the skip, jump or jogging element. Instead, just step or walk.

Aerobic workout

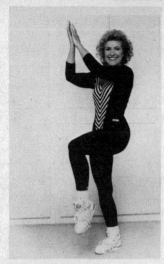 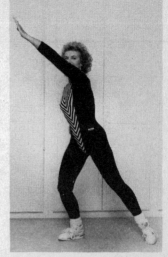

1 Step and clap
Raising and bending alternate knees, step from side to side clapping your hands above shoulder level. Repeat as many times as is comfortable and record your achievement each time you exercise. Increase the number of repetitions as you become fitter.

2 Lungeing
Swing one arm across and upwards at the same time as stepping out sideways with the corresponding leg (e.g. right arm/right leg). Repeat to the other side with the other arm reaching across and the other leg stepping out. Repeat as many times as possible without straining.

Aerobic workout

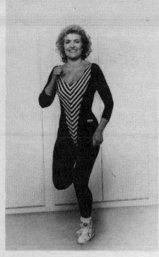 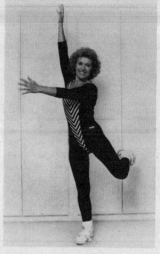

3 Jogging

Jog on the spot for as many steps as is comfortable. Record your achievement and try to increase the number of steps next time you exercise.

4 Swing and kick

Swing your arms first in front and then as high as possible to one side and at the same time allow the opposite leg to bend in a back-kick movement. Return the bent leg to the floor then swing your arms to the other side, lifting the other leg behind. Practise so that you get into the momentum of the exercise and repeat 16 times (8 to each side). As you become fitter you can skip as you do it. Record your progress each time you exercise.

Aerobic workout

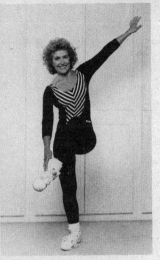 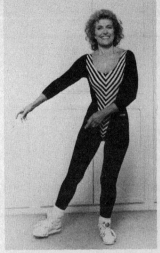

5 Alternate foot raises
Raise one foot towards the opposite hand and attempt a small jump as you do so. Repeat with the other foot and continue this skipping movement for as many times as you can without discomfort. Increase the number of repetitions as you become fitter.

6 Sideways jogging
Jog from side to side, allowing your arms to swing with you. Repeat as many times as possible and record the number of repetitions.

Aerobic workout

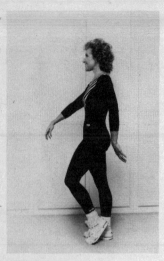 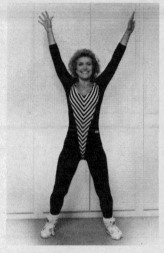

7 Walking jog
Walk on the spot, keeping your hands at a low level and repeat for 24 steps.

8 Jumping jacks
Stand with your feet together and your arms by your sides. Jump so that you land with your feet apart and your hands high. As you land on the floor ensure your knees bend over your ankles and not inwards. Jump again, lowering your hands to your sides and bringing your feet together into the starting position, bending your knees slightly as you land. This exercise should be performed rhythmically, jumping out and in, in time with the music. Repeat the movement as many times as you wish.

Aerobic workout

9 Half jack

For those who find jumping jacks uncomfortable, here is a low-impact alternative. Extend one leg out to the side and simultaneously raise both arms outwards at shoulder level. Bring the leg back to the centre, and at the same time lower your arms to your sides. Repeat the exercise as many times as you wish, alternating legs.

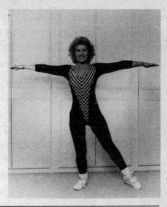

Muscular Strength and Endurance Exercises

Muscular strength and endurance exercises help our muscles to support our skeleton and maintain our posture and shape. It is these exercises that will particularly improve the shape of our hips and thighs. However, not only could they be harmful but they will not be as effective if we do not warm-up properly, so do not do them in isolation.

Strength exercises will obviously make our muscles stronger, whilst *Endurance* exercises enable the muscles to participate in continuous activity for longer. Both strength and endurance exercises improve our muscle tone.

To progress with *Strength* exercises we need to increase the resistance as we get fitter but to do only a few repetitions. We can increase the resistance by incorporating the use of a rubber band or a ball, thus making the muscle work harder. To progress in *Endurance* exercises we should increase the number of repetitions but keep the resistance low.

In the following exercises options are given for progressions which increase the level of difficulty of the exercises. The progressions are graded according to their level of difficulty. So, start with (a) and when you can perform this with ease, progress to (b) and so on. When you first begin these exercises do not start with the more difficult options unless you have previously exercised on a regular basis.

1 Outer thigh streamliner

Lie on your side in a straight line and prop your head on your hand as shown. Bend the lower leg to give you maximum balance. Bend the upper leg and then raise it up and down in a rhythmic movement and repeat 8 times initially, increasing the number of repetitions as you become fitter. It is preferable to perform sets of repetitions, thus allowing the muscle to rest in between and therefore achieving more repetitions ultimately. This can be done by rolling over and performing the exercise with the other leg and then returning to the initial side for the second set of repetitions. Keep your raised foot flexed and parallel with the floor throughout this exercise. Take care not to point the toes upwards, as to do so will cause the exercise to be ineffective. Your hips should remain level, one on top of the other.

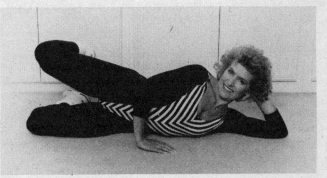

(a) Raise your bent upper leg no more than 24 ins (60 cm) up and down.

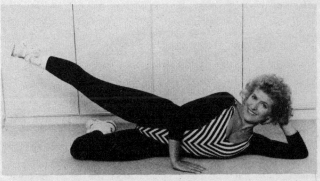

(b) Straighten your upper leg and raise it up and down.

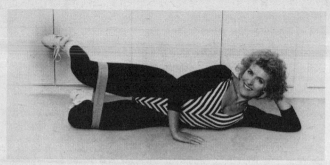

(c) Place a rubber band around your lower thighs. Keep your upper leg bent as you raise it up and down.

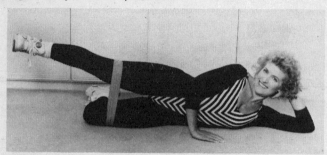

(d) With a band around your lower thighs, straighten your upper leg and raise it up and down.

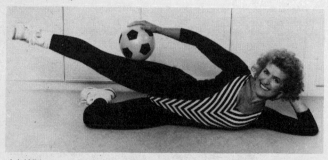

(e) With your upper leg straight, press against a ball to resist the movement as you raise the leg up and down. The harder you press the greater the resistance.

316

2 Inner thigh firmer

Remain lying on your side. The progressions of this exercise
gradually increase the degree of difficulty, thus making the exercise
even more effective as you become stronger. Again, start with
version (a) and try to increase your repetitions before moving on
to version (b) and so on. This exercise combines well with Exercise
1, working the inner and outer thighs on one side before rolling
over and repeating on the other side. You can perform sets of
repetitions of 8, 12 or 16, according to your ability, before rolling
over and repeating a second set. Increase the number of repetitions
as you become stronger. Because the range of movement of the
inner thigh is so restricted, this exercise can be performed at twice
the speed of that for the outer thigh. Pay special attention to the
position of your foot. Ensure your foot is parallel with the floor and
not pointing upwards when you lift the leg.

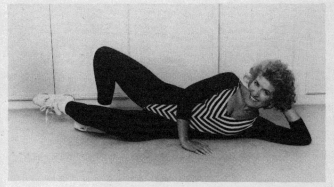

(a) Bend your upper leg and place the foot flat on the floor behind
the knee of your bent lower leg. Raise and lower bent (lower) leg.

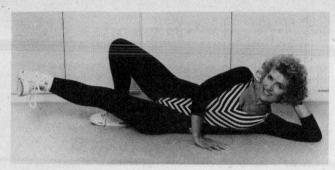

(b) Straighten your lower leg and raise it up and down.

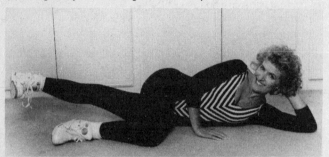

(c) With your upper leg dropped forwards, raise your straight lower leg up and down.

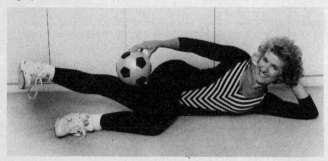

(d) Press a ball against the thigh of your lower leg as you raise the leg up and down. Increase the resistance by pressing harder with your hand.

3 Seat and thigh toner

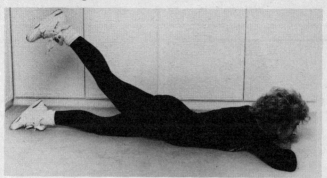

Lying face down, place your head on your hands. Raise one leg straight up and down, squeezing your buttocks as you do so. Repeat as many times as possible, then repeat with the other leg. Repeat the exercise again, alternating legs.

4 Thigh and buttock toner

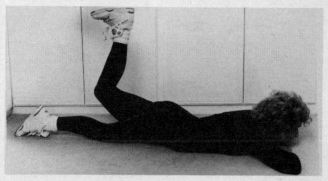

(a) Lie face down, with your head on your hands. Bend one leg, flex the foot and press its heel towards the ceiling, squeezing your buttocks as you do so. Repeat as many times as possible with one leg, then change legs and repeat. Change legs again and do another set of repetitions with each leg.

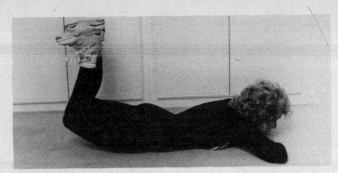

(b) Bend both legs and, with feet flexed, press both heels towards the ceiling. Repeat as many times as you can.

5 *Back thigh toner*

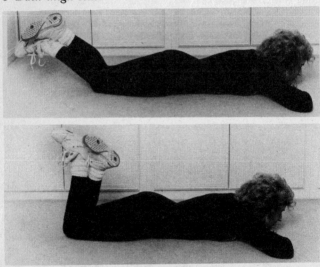

Lying face down, with your head on your hands, bend both legs and place one foot behind the other. Raise and lower your feet, pressing your legs against each other at the ankles, resisting the raising and lowering. For maximum benefit, squeeze your buttocks together as you raise and lower the legs. Change legs and repeat with the other leg on top. Continue the up and down movement for a similar number of repetitions. If possible, repeat the whole exercise again.

6 Inner thigh toner

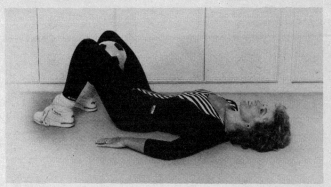

Lie on your back, bending your knees. Place a football between your inner thighs and squeeze your legs together as many times as possible. Adjust the position of the ball to achieve maximum effect (you'll feel which is the hardest position). Proceed to the Front thigh tightener and then return and repeat this Inner thigh toner.

7 Front thigh tightener

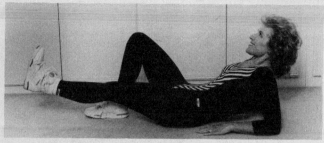

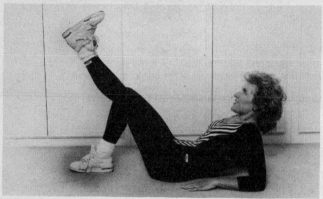

Lying with both knees bent and feet flat on the floor, straighten and then raise one leg up and down 16 times. Change legs and repeat. Repeat with each leg again. Increase the number of sets as you become fitter. It is important that the static leg remains bent. For maximum benefit, the working leg should not be raised beyond the height of the knee of the bent leg. Now return to the Inner thigh toner and do 2 sets of repetitions of both exercises.

8 Outer thigh toner

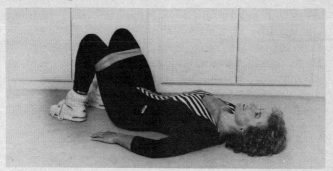

Place a rubber band around your lower thighs, lie on the floor and bend your knees. Make sure the band is short enough to be taut, without the knees being too far apart. Then, alternately widen and narrow the gap between your knees, at the same time resisting against the band. Perform the maximum number of repetitions you can do reasonably comfortably. Rest for 30 seconds and then do another set of repetitions.

Stretches

After we have worked our muscles hard through the aerobic and muscular strength and endurance exercises we need to stretch them out again to return them to their normal state. It is also important to encourage our muscles to be used in an extended form as well as in a contraction. Otherwise bad posture could result, with long-term detrimental effects to our body shape.

Some stretches should be held in the extreme position for a minimum of 6 to 8 seconds; others can be held for longer and even progressed still further. This second group are called developmental stretches.

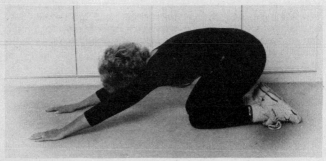

1 Seat stretch
Position yourself on your hands and knees and slowly lean back towards your feet without allowing your seat to rest on your heels. Stretch out your arms as far as possible and enjoy the beautiful stretch throughout your body. Hold the extreme position for 10 seconds then relax.

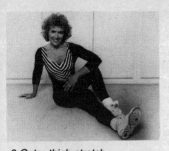 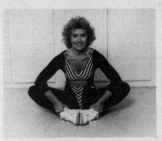

2 Outer thigh stretch
Sit with your legs outstretched in front of you. Place your right foot on the left side of your left leg, your right hand on the floor and your left elbow on the right side of your right knee. Your left hand is on your right thigh. Using your left elbow, ease your right knee across your body and feel the stretch in your outer thigh. Hold for 8 seconds, then relax. Repeat the exercise with your left leg over and using your right elbow to ease your left knee across.

3 Inner thigh stretch
Sitting with soles of your feet placed together, rest your elbows against your knees. Keeping your back straight, try to ease your knees down without straining. Hold for 10 seconds and then try to ease your knees down a little further and hold for another 10 seconds. Slowly relax.

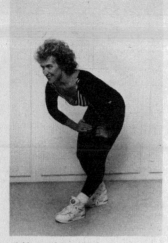

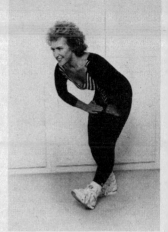

4 Hamstring stretch
Stand with one foot behind the other and your feet hip-width apart, feet pointing straight ahead. Keep the front leg straight and bend the back leg, lowering your hips. Place your hands on your thighs (not on your knees) and hold for 15 seconds. Proceed to the next exercise.

5 Calf stretch
Maintaining the position of the Hamstring stretch, raise the toes of your front foot, keeping your front leg straight and your heel on the floor. Hold for a count of 15. Relax and then repeat Exercises 4 and 5 with the other leg forward.

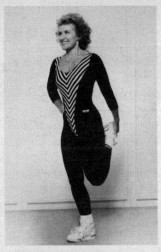

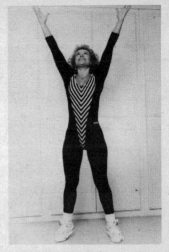

6 Front thigh stretch
Standing with your feet together, bend your left leg and take hold of the foot with your left hand. Stretch the front thigh muscles by easing your foot as close to your seat as possible. Do not strain. Hold the position for 6 seconds before slowly releasing the leg to the floor. Repeat with your right leg.

7 Whole body stretch
Stand up straight, raise up on to the balls of your feet and stretch up towards the ceiling. Stretch your whole body from your fingers to your toes and feel revitalized.

12
Cellulite:
Do the various treatments help?

Anyone who says cellulite doesn't exist obviously doesn't have it and never has had it. I *have* had it – in vast quantities – and still have some. To me there is absolutely no doubt whatsoever that cellulite exists. It is fat, but it is different in its composition in so far as it gives the skin an ugly and uneven appearance. It is usually found round the thighs, the hips and the upper arms of women. Men rarely have it.

The respondents who completed my questionnaire were asked if the incidence of cellulite had reduced as a result of following my diet. There was absolutely no doubt from the response I received that a dramatic improvement had been enjoyed.

I am yet to be convinced that massage creams for cellulite are really effective. It may simply be that in applying the cream the physical action of massaging does the trick, as one of the reasons for the creation of cellulite is poor circulation. Any sort of massage is obviously going to encourage a better flow of blood and oxygen.

Recent research has established that aerobic exercise really can act as a 'fat burner'. However, the activity needs to be sustained for a minimum of twenty minutes, which is quite a lot to ask of most

328

people. It is, though, something that we can aim to achieve as we get fitter.

Let us discuss *cellulite* in more detail and see why and how these treatments can help us.

Cellulite is a modified form of fat tissue found just below the surface of the skin. It all begins with the stagnation of the blood in capillaries (tiny blood vessels), and this leads to a flow of blood fluids (plasma) through the capillary walls which separate fat-storing cells known as adipose cells. Small groups of these cells become surrounded by collagen fibre bundles in what are known as micronodules. These in turn group together to form macronodules which are responsible for the skin's irregular, wrinkled appearance. It is this uneven appearance that distinguishes cellulite from neighbouring fat on the tummy or waist which is almost always relatively smooth and uniform.

Our bodies use these fat cells and the connective tissue as a kind of storehouse for waste products and because these particular fat cells are metabolically less active than other cells in the body they make an ideal location for whatever toxic waste products the body would like to keep out of the way so that they don't pollute the bloodstream. It is easy to see, therefore, that the problem is a particularly difficult one to solve as the area is partially 'cut off' from our normal circulation.

Consequently these areas are the first to exhibit extra fat and the last to actually reduce.

Dietary factors play an important part in our battle with cellulite. A diet high in fresh fruit and vegetables is obviously to be recommended as it encourages digestion and elimination. These are also

329

very healthy foods rich in vitamins and minerals. Wholegrain cereals are good for the same reasons, and protein foods (meat, fish, low-fat cheese) balance the diet and give all the necessary nutrients. Skimmed milk and low-fat spreads should also be preferred to the full-fat equivalents in the family diet. Foods high in sugar, salt, fat and spices should be kept to a minimum, and the consumption of alcohol should be restricted, too, though there is no need to eliminate it – one drink a day is acceptable.

Toning tables: In recent years toning tables have grown widely in popularity and the promise of a trimmer body without actually working for it has attracted many to try them. These machines are cleverly designed to work the muscles in your body without you moving from the bed that creates all the movements. There is little doubt that these machines do work the muscles, but the most important muscle of all, the heart, gets no exercise at all.

As I said earlier, we cannot turn fat into muscle, so toned muscle still covered in fat will continue to give an unattractive appearance. Without wishing to be negative, or discouraging, in all honesty I feel I cannot recommend anyone to follow this line of treatment. Not only is it extremely boring and, because of the expense, an unlikely means of exercising in the long term, it is certainly not going to make you fitter over all. Just as we need to re-educate our palate towards sensible eating in order to maintain our new leaner figure in the long term, so we need to find a form of exercise that we enjoy and that we will continue throughout our life.

Passive exercise machines: A passive exercise machine

also exercises muscles while you lie on a couch or bed. A portable machine running on batteries is available, or a larger electrically powered 'salon' model. Both come supplied with full instructions for correct usage.

The portable machine consists of an operating unit plus eight plastic-covered wires which in turn are connected to round rubber pads. The pads are placed at strategic points on your body (depending on which part you wish to tone), and are held in place with wide elasticated bands. The machine works on the body through an electric pulsing current which activates the muscles you wish to tone without physical movement. Your legs may *feel* like they have walked thirty miles at the end of your forty-minute session, but you won't have sore feet or feel at all tired!

This all sounds too good to be true, but there are certain disadvantages. The machines are not cheap, and are very time-consuming. They are extremely inconvenient if someone calls unexpectedly at your door!

No passive exercise machine will eliminate fat. You can only do that by reducing your energy input by calorie cutting and increasing your energy output by taking aerobic exercise. However they can help your muscle shape, and they will certainly make your long-lost muscles come back to life, so if for any reason you can't take normal exercise, a machine could be invaluable to you. For some people they work very well, but not everyone can tolerate the strange sensation given out by some of these machines.

So, to sum up, the answer must be a firm 'yes' to

exercise. Anything that makes your heart work harder and exercises your muscles will help to reduce the amount of fat on your body by burning up extra calories. We will become fitter and generally healthier by such activities. There is no easy cure for cellulite, though undoubtedly a low-fat diet is one of the most effective ways of reducing it. Consistent aerobic exercise will also help. **Massage creams** are comparatively ineffective and can be expensive, as are **toning tables** and **passive exercise machines**. What it all boils down to is this: we don't need to spend any extra money; we must simply *eat healthily* and *get moving*.

13
The Maintenance Programme

Losing weight is ironically always the easiest part of weight control partly because of the novelty value and partly because the instructions that we have to follow are quite clear. The problems arise once we *stop* dieting. Suddenly we feel free from the restrictions that have been placed upon us and it is all too easy to think, 'Great. I can now eat chocolate, chips and cakes!' In this respect the Hip and Thigh Diet is more helpful, because you cannot return to eating lots of the foods that made you fat in the first place – that is, if you want to keep your new slimmer and trimmer figure. But you *can* relax a little and you *can* eat a wider variety of foods, including more eggs, low-fat hard cheeses and fatless cakes – in fact almost anything you like as long as it is low in fat.

On most diets the metabolic rate falls because the body adjusts to a reduced calorie intake and when people return to 'normal' eating the weight piles back on even though they are not over-eating. It all seems so unfair doesn't it? Fortunately, because the Hip and Thigh Diet offers so much food – more calories than most diets would allow – the metabolic rate hardly falls at all. This is particularly evident with those who undertake regular exercise.

We lose weight when we consume fewer calories

than our body needs, and we therefore make up the deficit from our stores of fat. After reaching our desired weight, we need to feed our body sufficient calories to maintain that new weight, but not ruin all our good work by eating too much and storing the remainder as fat again. It is a tricky situation, but so long as you keep a careful eye on the tape measure and the scales, you will soon become more confident in your ability to keep your weight constant. If you do over-indulge and you do gain weight, by returning to the diet for a few days you should be able to undo the damage quite quickly. But, if you wish to retain your slimmer hips and thighs, you must realize that a low-fat diet in the long term is essential. I don't think you need to worry too much with this point, however, as so many of my correspondents stated that their taste buds had been completely re-educated after following the diet – as were my own – and it was no effort at all to maintain their new figures. Many in fact completed questionnaires after they had been on the Maintenance Programme and they commented that with previous diets they had always regained the lost weight very quickly, but this time it was quite a different story. I could sense they were confident that they would never return to their bad, high-fat, eating habits ever again.

With all this in mind it is clear that this chapter is a very important one. It is vital to learn which foods may be eaten freely and which should be avoided so that we can have slim hips and thighs for ever!

You may prefer to release yourself from the restrictions of an actual diet. If so, please read carefully the following four pages. They explain your nutritional requirements and which foods may be reintroduced into your daily diet, together with those which should still be avoided.

There is no need to tot up your daily intake of grams of fat. If you follow the basic principles already learned whilst on the diet, you really have nothing to fear. It is only when you start breaking the rules about forbidden foods on a regular basis that you will undo the good results that you have achieved. The very fact that we have avoided the need to count any form of units or calories throughout the diet has weaned us away from this negative habit. It would be a shame to start now with the counting of grams of fat. So relax and just remember what you've learned so far.

The following lists of foods and recommendations should form the pattern of foods consumed for a healthy diet. A daily diet made up of reasonable quantities from each category will ensure a balanced consumption of essential nutrients to maintain health and energy, without including unnecessary foods which add useless calories and lead to unwanted fat. A diet which follows these recommendations will encourage a healthy digestion, and constipation problems will become a thing of the past.

Protein and minerals

A minimum of 6 oz (175 g) of meat, fish, eggs or cheese should be consumed daily.

½ pint (250 ml) skimmed or semi-skimmed milk should be consumed daily – maximum 1 pint (500 ml) per day.

Fish	Any type	Steamed, grilled or microwaved without fat
Meat	Any type, lean cuts only	Grilled, roast or microwaved, without fat, and with all fat trimmed off before cooking, or trimmed afterwards
Poultry	Any type	Grilled, roast or microwaved, without fat. Do not eat any skin or fat
Offal	Any type	Steamed, baked or microwaved, without fat
Eggs		Cook in any way without the use of fat. Consume no more than 2 per week
Cheese	Preferably low-fat Cheddar or Edam	Restrict to 4 oz (100 g) per week if possible
Cheese	Cottage	Unlimited quantities may be consumed
Yogurt, fromage frais, Quark	Any type	Unlimited

Vitamins

Approx. 12 oz (350 g) of fruit or vegetables should be consumed daily.

Vegetables	Any type	Unlimited, but always without butter
Fruit	Any type	Unlimited. Serve on its own, or with yogurt, fromage frais, Quark or non-Cornish ice cream

Carbohydrates
A minimum of 4 oz (100 g) to be consumed daily.

Bread	Wholemeal or Crispbreads	Unlimited if eaten without fat; otherwise limit consumption to 3 slices of bread a day or 8 rye crispbreads
Cereal	Breakfast	1–2 oz (25–50 g) per day
Rice	Brown	2–3 oz (50–75 g) per day
Pasta	Fat free	Average portions 2–3 oz (50–75 g)
Potatoes	Boiled or baked	Unlimited if eaten without fat

Fats
Consume as little as possible.

Low fat spread	Any brand	Maximum of ½ oz (12 g) per day only. No butter or margarine
Cream	Single	1 oz (25 g) very occasionally

In addition, the following foods may be eaten in moderation
Milk puddings made with skimmed milk
Reduced-oil salad dressings
Cakes made without fat (see recipes for Apple Gâteau, pages 277–8, Kim's Cake, pages 275–6, Banana and Sultana Cake, page 276)
Ice cream (non-Cornish variety)
Pancakes made with skimmed milk
Yorkshire pudding made with skimmed milk in non-stick baking tin and no added fat

Trifle made with only fatless sponge and custard made with skimmed milk, no cream

Cauliflower cheese made with low-fat cheese and skimmed milk

Sausages – low-fat brands, if grilled well

Nuts – only very few and avoid Brazils, Barcelona nuts or almonds

Horlicks, Ovaltine or drinking chocolate

Sauces if possible made with skimmed milk, but *no* butter

Soups excepting cream soups

Soya

Continue to avoid the following foods

Butter, margarine

Oil, lard, dripping, etc.

Fried bread

Chapatis made with fat

Biscuits, all sweet varieties

Cakes, all except fat-free recipes

Milk, dried, and Gold Top

Cream, double, whipping, sterilized, canned

Cheese, all types except Edam, cottage, low-fat Cheddar

Cheese spread

Quiches, Scotch eggs, cheese soufflé, Welsh Rarebit, etc.

Fat from meat, streaky bacon

Skin from chicken, turkey, duck, goose, etc.

Salami, pâté, pork pie, meat pies, etc.

Sprats or whitebait, fried

Fish in oil

Anything fried, including mushrooms or onions

Desiccated coconut

Brazil nuts, almonds, Barcelona nuts

Chocolate, toffees, fudge, caramel, butterscotch
Mayonnaise
Marzipan
French dressing made with oil
Pastries
Pork scratchings
Avocados

Drinks

Tea and coffee may be drunk freely if drunk black, or may be drunk white using skimmed or semi-skimmed milk. Use artificial sweetener whenever possible, though on the Maintenance programme a little sugar may be taken.

Unless otherwise stated in the menus, your alcohol allowance of one drink per day (2 for men) remains unchanged but drinks may be 'saved up' as required. One drink means a single measure of any spirits, a glass of wine, or small glass of sherry or half a pint of beer or lager. Low calorie mixers and diet drinks should be used whenever possible and these may be drunk freely.

You may drink as much water as you like.

Grape, apple, unsweetened orange, grapefruit, pineapple, exotic fruit juices may be drunk in moderation. The recipes for low-calorie drinks detailed on pages 285–8 are still ideal for the Maintenance programme.

Sauces, gravy, spreads and dressings

Sauces made without fat, and with low-fat skimmed milk from the daily allowance, may be eaten. Thicker gravy made with gravy powder or low-fat granules may also be served with main courses. Vegemite or Bovril may be used freely to add flavour to cooking and on bread. For salads select any of the fat-free dressings (see recipes). You can have the Seafood Dressing and Reduced-oil Dressing as desired.

Anyone who has been following the Hip and Thigh Diet for some time will be very familiar with the types of meals that can be eaten. Now that you have reached the Maintenance stage, you can simply either increase the amounts of foods allowed previously or add additional foods to your menus. As this is going to be the way you are going to eat for the rest of your life, it is important that you begin educating yourself into long-term habits. You will soon find from the tape measure and the scales how far you can go and you will be able to judge when that little extra is too much as far as your own metabolic rate is concerned. I have stayed on the Maintenance programme for six years now and find that, provided I stick always to low-fat eating, I am able to maintain my weight. As soon as I start eating fat, sometimes unintentionally, the weight goes on frighteningly quickly. However, I have come to terms with the fact that I can eat very well if I eat low-fat and so there is little sacrifice to be made.

Just remind yourself often that you've worked very hard to achieve the size and shape that you are now; it would be a dreadful shame to go back to your old eating habits and to waste all that effort. If you want to be slim in the future you have to stick to the basic rules. The less you cheat with high-fat foods the easier you'll find it is to maintain, and to become more relaxed about, your eating habits.

Whatever you do, don't get into the habit of eating fat again. Whether it be butter or margarine on your bread or eating high-fat cheese with biscuits, you will find yourself on a desperately slippery slope. It doesn't take long to get back the taste for fatty food that you have worked so hard to be rid of. Don't try it and then you won't miss it. Although some people find that they are repulsed by the taste of fatty food after they have been on a low-fat diet, others soon find it attractive again. Please do not take the risk.

To put it in a nutshell: on the Maintenance programme eat what you like, but eat low-fat. See how you get on and watch your progress. If you find your weight and your measurements get out of hand, then return to the Diet until you are back at your goal weight once more. Then proceed with caution, gradually increasing one or two extra foods when you feel confident to do so.

I would also recommend that anyone who reaches his or her goal writes a personal statement that day. Date it and write: how you think you look in the mirror; what the scales say; what your measurements are; and how much better you feel as a result of having shed those extra pounds. Then record some of the memories: how horrible you used to feel when you were overweight (perhaps including here an unkind comment from someone); how you felt when you went to buy clothes; and what it used to be like when you had to exert yourself either to run in an emergency or when you were just going about your everyday work. You do not need to show this record to anyone – keep it safely tucked away in a drawer and take it out occasionally just to remind yourself how good it is being slim. Also, make sure that you hang on to one item of large clothing as a reminder of how much weight you've lost. Never throw this garment away. Similarly, do not throw away all the old photographs of the former fat you. Keep them to remind yourself vividly what you've left behind. As we become accustomed to being slimmer, sometimes we forget just how big we used to be and we are self-critical of a still less-than-perfect shape. We need reminders such as old clothing or photographs to jolt us back to reality and to encourage us to enjoy our great achievements.

14
Living life to the full

Overweight can cause us to have such a low opinion of ourselves that we can easily lose out on our true potential. We learned in an earlier chapter how some of my slimmers had found confidence to embark on a new life after acquiring a new figure – one with which they felt happy – and surely this must be true of everyone.

I believe we all have a talent. For some it may be flower arranging or decorating, others may find they are a dab hand at organizing, some may have a flair in business or writing poetry, sewing or knitting, teaching, communicating or supporting – a million and one options to choose from! Your talent may be obvious to you already but, as yet, you haven't had the courage to develop it properly – or perhaps you fancy having a go at something but so far just haven't had the nerve.

With a new, happy and healthy attitude to life, now is the time to give it a try. You may decide to book into your local night school, start taking driving lessons, go back to work or start a business. Until you try you'll have no idea of your natural ability and you *could* be brilliantly successful. If you *don't* try you won't ever know and as someone very wisely put it, 'You get paid for doing, not dreaming.' So don't just sit about thinking about it – do it! Get rid of excuses and eliminate from your vocabulary the words 'I can't'. And as the old saying goes, 'If at first you don't succeed, try, try again.' If you try hard enough you are almost bound to succeed.

If we aren't happy with ourselves we will *never* realize our true potential and then we *will* feel a failure, so when those people who *don't* have a weight problem criticize those of us who do and who try to lose weight, I don't think they realize how important it is psychologically for us to feel happy about ourselves. A slim body is very important indeed to some people – we must accept that. Paradoxically it is those of us who suffer with a weight problem who desperately *need* to be slim. Those who are naturally slim just don't understand how we feel.

When we have more confidence we are able to sort out our lives – those problems that previously we felt unable to solve. Many who are basically unhappy put up with that unhappiness for years just because they lack self-confidence. In my talks I describe life as a garden. Our garden of life can be full of flowers or full of weeds and if we are to achieve real happiness we should remove the 'weeds' one by one and replace them with flowers. Perhaps the problem might be a selfish next-door neighbour; a boss who you feel hates you, so that you dread going to work; a relative who really gets you down or a job that you loathe. Whatever it is, it won't get better unless you do something about it.

When we have more confidence we can stand up to people so much better, and make our own views known. Most of the time the person who is actually getting on our nerves has absolutely no idea that there *is* a problem at all. So, the sooner we can discuss it the better! We shouldn't use bulldozer tactics to clear away the weeds, because if we do we will hurt people and that's the *last* thing we want to do. But by thoughtfully putting our point across – as soon as possible – you'd be amazed how understanding and co-operative people can be.

Aggression is often displayed as a compensation for a lack of confidence. As soon as you become polite and charming – though it must of course be sincere – the world becomes a most wonderful place in which to live. I try to build up the confidence of anyone I can. When slimmers have been coming to my classes for a few weeks, I begin to see a flower blossoming. Sometimes they start exercising in a tracksuit but later on, when they have lost some weight, they have the confidence to wear a leotard. I try to make a point of saying how much slimmer they look – I can *see* when they've lost weight. When I tell them, they are positively thrilled and they are like a flower growing. It is beautiful to see.

We all love to receive compliments, but oh, the joy of *giving* them. If you have the confidence to compliment people, you will find everyone is so friendly. So I believe it is a very good thing to get into the habit of complimenting people. And if you are fortunate enough to be on the receiving end, do accept the compliment as if it were a gift – graciously and with gratitude. Don't shrug it off. When you have lost all those inches on the Hip and Thigh Diet and someone says, 'You look fantastic,' please say 'Thank you!' and enjoy it!

15
A guide to fat in food – the complete tables

The following tables list the average fat content of everyday foods which are available in shops or served in restaurants, and illustrate, at a glance, the fat content for easy reading and learning.

The tables do not include the fat content of the recipes included in this book. These recipes have been carefully designed to use as little fat as possible and are therefore considerably lower in fat content in comparison with 'standard recipes'.

By comparing suggested meals listed in Chapter 8, alternative meals may be designed to suit your own individual tastes, bearing in mind the fat content of the various foods. Some foods, of course, are low in fat but high in calories, so a certain amount of common sense is needed to ensure that you do not overeat and gain weight. For instance alcohol and boiled sweets contain no fat, but they contain loads of calories, so their consumption should be moderated! And do bear in mind the foods that are high in fat but consumed in very small quantities, e.g., mustard and curry powder. Mind you, I doubt you would be able to eat enough of these to damage your figure without blowing your head off!

As a rule of thumb for those following the Maintenance programme, try to select foods from the tables which have a fat content of not more than 3 grams per ounce.

The food tables have been drawn up to indicate the fat content of 25 grams of each item listed and for the sake of convenience I have taken 25 grams to equal one ounce instead of the actual equivalent of 28.349 grams to the ounce. The reason for this is that most products are labelled with the composition per 100 grams and my tables are therefore based on a quarter of this value.

By reading these tables you will learn quickly which foods are high and which are low in fat and after a while you will be able to steer an easy course to healthy eating and a long and active life.

FAT TABLES

Grams per 25g/1oz (approx)

	1	2	3	4	5	6	7	8	9	10	11	12	13	14	15	16	17	18	19	20	21	22	23	24	25

ALCOHOL

Beers:

Brown Ale		•
Canned Beer		•
Draught		•
Keg		•
Lager		•
Pale Ale		•
Stout		•
Stout, Extra		•
Strong Ale		•

Ciders:

| All types | | • |

Wines:

| All types | | | • |

Wines, Fortified:

| Port | | | | • |
| Sherry | | | • |

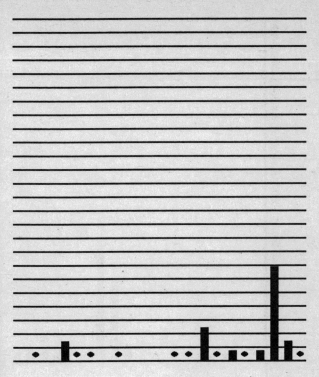

Vermouths:
   All types
Liqueurs:
   Advocaat
   Cherry Brandy
   Curacao
Spirits:
   All types

BAKING PRODUCTS AND
SEASONINGS

Baking Powder
Bovril
Curry Powder
Gelatine
Ginger, Ground
Marmite
Oxo Cubes
Mustard Powder
Pepper
Salt

♦ = negligible

Grams per 25g/1oz (approx)

Scale: 1 2 3 4 5 6 7 8 9 10 11 12 13 14 15 16 17 18 19 20 21 22 23 24 25

Vinegar
Yeast, Baker's
Yeast, Dried

BEANS
Baked Beans
Red Kidney Beans

BEVERAGES
Bournvita
Cocoa Powder
Coffee Whitener
Coffee and Chicory Essence
Coffee
Drinking Chocolate
Horlicks
Ovaltine
Tea

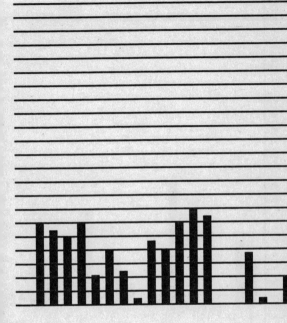

BISCUITS – SWEET
Chocolate, full coated
Cream Biscuits
Digestive, Plain
Digestive, Chocolate
Garibaldi
Ginger Nuts
Jaffa Cakes
Matzo
Muesli Biscuits
Semi-Sweet
Short-Sweet
Shortbread
Wafers, Filled

BISCUITS – SAVOURY
Cream Crackers
Crispbread, Rye
Crispbread, Wheat Starch
        Reduced
Oatcakes

♦ = negligible

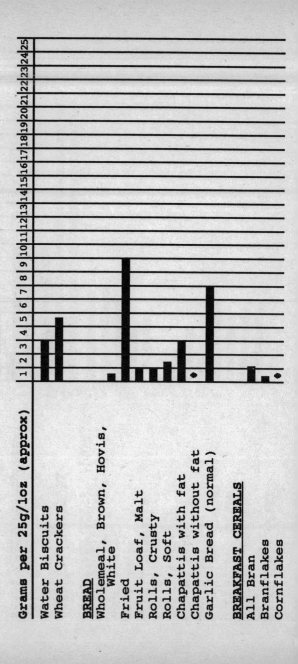

Grapenuts
Muesli
Oatmeal, raw
Porridge
Puffed Wheat
Ready Brek
Rice Krispies
Rye and Raisin
Shredded Wheat
Special K
Sugar Puffs
Weetabix

BUTTER AND BUTTER SUBSTITUTES

Butter
Flora
Gold
Gold Lowest
Shape Sunflower Spread

◆ = negligible

Grams per 25g/1oz (approx)

CAKES AND PASTRIES

Scale: 1 2 3 4 5 6 7 8 9 10 11 12 13 14 15 16 17 18 19 20 21 22 23 24 25

Item	Approx. grams per 25g/1oz
Cheesecake	4
Currant Buns	2
Doughnuts	4
Eclairs	6
Fancy, Iced	4
Fruit, Rich	3
Gingerbread	3
Jam Tarts	1
Madeira	4
Mince Pies	2
Pastry, Choux	5
Pastry, Flaky	10
Pastry, Shortcrust	8
Plain	3
Rock	4
Scones	3
Scotch Pancakes	4
Sponge with fat	7

Sponge without fat

CHEESE
Camembert
Cheddar
Low Fat White and Coloured
Cheddar
Ordinary Mature Cheddar
Vegetarian Cheddar
Low Fat Cheshire
Ordinary Cheshire
Danish Blue
Edam
Double Gloucester
Gouda
Gruyere
Red Leicester
Lymeswold
Parmesan
Stilton
Cottage with Cream

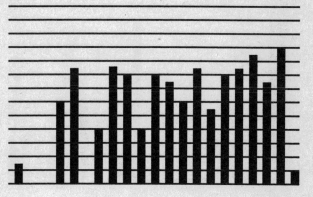

◆ = negligible

Grams per 25g/1oz (approx)

	Grams per 25g/1oz (approx)
Low Fat Cottage Cheese – Plain	1
Low Fat Cottage Cheeses:	
Cottage Cheese with Pineapple	1
with Onion and Chives	1
with Caribbean Fruit	1
Mexican Style	1
Italian Style	1
Cream Cheese	12
Low Fat Soft Cheese	2
Plain or with Chives, Pineapple etc	2
Cheese Spread	5
CONDIMENTS	
Apple Sauce	•
Cranberry Sauce	•
English Mustard	2

(Horizontal axis scale: 1 2 3 4 5 6 7 8 9 10 11 12 13 14 15 16 17 18 19 20 21 22 23 24 25)

Horseradish Sauce
Redcurrant Jelly
Tartare Sauce

CONFECTIONERY
Boiled Sweets

Chocolate, average, Milk or
    Plain

Chocolate, Fancy and Filled
Chocolate, Nut and Raisin
Bounty Bar
Mars Bar
Fruit Gums
Fudge
Humbugs
Liquorice
Pastilles
Peppermints
Toffees

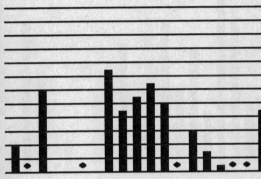

◆ - negligible

Grams per 25g/1oz (approx)

CREAM AND CREAM SUBSTITUTES

Food	Grams per 25g/1oz (approx)
Cream, Single	5
Cream, Double	12
Cream, Cornish Clotted	15
Cream, Soured	5
Cream, Whipping	8
Cream, Sterilised Canned	6
Dream Topping	11

CRISPS AND SNACKS

Food	Grams per 25g/1oz (approx)
Potato Crisps	9
Low Fat Crisps	7

EGGS

Food	Grams per 25g/1oz (approx)
Whole, Raw	3
White Only	0
Yolk Only	7
Dried	11
Boiled	3

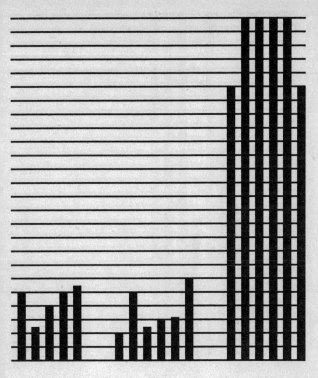

Fried
Poached
Omelette
Scotch Egg
Scrambled

EGG AND CHEESE DISHES
Cauliflower Cheese
Cheese Soufflé
Macaroni Cheese
Pizza, Cheese and Tomato
Quiche
Welsh Rarebit

FATS AND OILS
Butter
Coconut Oil
Cod liver Oil
Compound Cooking Fat
Dripping, Beef
Flora

◆ = negligible

Grams per 25g/1oz (approx)

Food	Grams per 25g/1oz (approx)
Gold Lowest	6
Lard	25
Low Fat Spread	9
Margarine, all kinds	25
Olive Oil	25
Low Fat Sunflower Spread	9
Suet, Block	25
Suet, Shredded	22
Vegetable Oils	25
FISH — Fatty Fish	
Eel, Stewed	3
Herring, Fried	4
Herring, Grilled	3
Bloater, Grilled	5
Kipper, Baked	2
Mackerel, Fried	2
Pilchards in Tomato Sauce	1
Salmon, Steamed	4

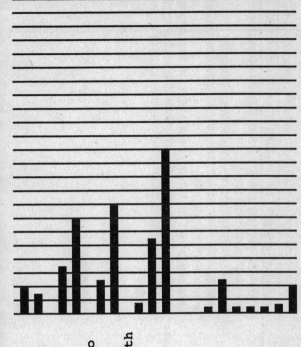

Salmon, Canned
Salmon, Smoked
Sardines, Canned in Oil
    (fish only)
Sardines, Fish plus Oil
Sardines, Canned in Tomato
    Sauce
Sprats, Fried with Bones
Trout, (Brown) Steamed with
    Bones
Tuna
Whitebait, Fried

FISH — White Fish
Cod, Baked
Cod, Fried in Batter
Cod, Grilled
Cod, Poached
Cod, Steamed
Cod, Smoked, Poached
Haddock, Fried

♦ = negligible

Grams per 25g/1oz (approx)	1	2	3	4	5	6	7	8	9	10	11	12	13	14	15	16	17	18	19	20	21	22	23	24	25
Haddock, Steamed																									
Haddock, Smoked, Steamed																									
Halibut, Steamed																									
Lemon sole, Fried																									
Lemon Sole, Steamed																									
Plaice, Fried in Batter																									
Plaice, Fried in Breadcrumbs																									
Plaice, Steamed																									
Whiting, Fried																									
Whiting, Steamed																									
FISH - Other Seafood																									
Dogfish, Fried in Batter																									
Skate, Fried in Batter																									
Crab, Boiled																									
Crab, Boiled, weighed with shell																									
Lobster, Boiled																									

Lobster, Boiled, weighed
with shell
Prawns, Boiled
Prawns, Boiled, weighed with
shell
Scampi, Fried
Shrimps, Boiled
Shrimps, Boiled with shells
Shrimps, Canned
Cockles, Boiled
Mussels, Boiled
Oysters, Raw
Scallops, Steamed
Whelks, Boiled
Winkles
Roe, (cod hard) Fried
Roe, (herring soft) Fried

FLOUR
Cornflour
Custard Powder

♦ = negligible

Grams per 25g/1oz (approx)

Food	Grams per 25g/1oz (approx)
Flour, Wholemeal	1
Flour, White, etc.	1
FROMAGE FRAIS	
Ordinary Fromage Frais	2
Low Fat Fromage Frais	•
Low Fat Apricot Fromage Frais	
Low Fat Strawberry Fromage Frais	
Low Fat Orange Fromage Frais	
Low Fat Raspberry Fromage Frais	
FRUIT	
Apples	•
Apricots	•
Avocado Pears	5
Bananas	•
Bilberries	•

Blackberries

Cherries

Cherries, Glacé

Coconut – Flesh only

Coconut – Milk only

Cranberries

Currants

Damsons

Dates

Figs

Fruit Pie Filling

Fruit Salad

Gooseberries

Grapes

Grapefruit

Greengages

Guavas

Lemons

Loganberries

Lychees

Mandarin Oranges

♦ = negligible

Grams per 25g/1oz (approx)

	1	2	3	4	5	6	7	8	9	10	11	12	13	14	15	16	17	18	19	20	21	22	23	24	25
Mangoes																									
Medlars																									
Melons																									
Mulberries																									
Nectarines																									
Olives																									
Oranges																									
Passion Fruit																									
Paw Paw																									
Peaches																									
Pears																									
Pineapple																									
Plums																									
Pomegranate																									
Prunes																									
Quinces																									
Raisins																									
Raspberries																									
Rhubarb																									

Strawberries
Sultanas
Tangerines

GAME

Grouse, Roast weighed with bone

Partridge:
    Roast
    Roast, weighed with bone

Pheasant:
    Roast
    Roast, weighed with bone

Pigeon:
    Roast
    Roast, weighed with bone

Hare:
    Stewed
    Stewed weighed with bone

 = negligible

Grams per 25g/1oz (approx)

	1	2	3	4	5	6	7	8	9	10	11	12	13	14	15	16	17	18	19	20	21	22	23	24	25

Rabbit:
  Stewed
  Stewed weighed with bone
Venison, Roast

GRAINS
Barley, Pearl
Bran
Rye
Sago
Semolina
Tapioca, raw

GRAVY PRODUCTS - DRY
Gravy Granules
Gravy Powder

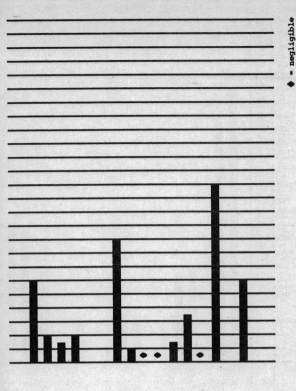

ICE CREAM
Choc Ice
Cornish Dairy
Vanilla Plain
Vanilla Soft Scoop

JAMS AND PRESERVES
Chocolate Spread
Honeycomb
Honey in jars
Jam
Lemon Curd, Starch Based
Lemon Curd, Home Made
Marmalade
Peanut Butter

MARZIPAN

MEAT

◆ = negligible

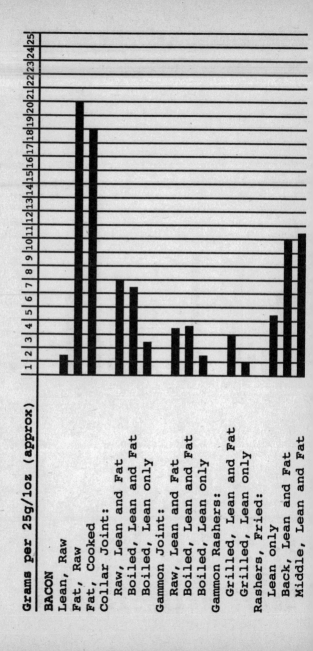

Grams per 25g/1oz (approx)

BACON
Lean, Raw
Fat, Raw
Fat, Cooked
Collar Joint:
  Raw, Lean and Fat
  Boiled, Lean and Fat
  Boiled, Lean only
Gammon Joint:
  Raw, Lean and Fat
  Boiled, Lean and Fat
  Boiled, Lean only
Gammon Rashers:
  Grilled, Lean and Fat
  Grilled, Lean only
Rashers, Fried:
  Lean only
  Back, Lean and Fat
  Middle, Lean and Fat

1 2 3 4 5 6 7 8 9 10 11 12 13 14 15 16 17 18 19 20 21 22 23 24 25

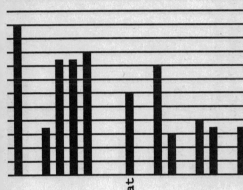

Streaky, Lean and Fat
Rashers, Grilled:
  Lean only
  Back, Lean and Fat
  Middle, Lean and Fat
  Streaky, Lean and Fat

BEEF
Brisket, Boiled, Lean and Fat
Forerib Roast:
  Lean and Fat
  Lean only
Mince:
  Raw
  Stewed
Rump Steak, Fried:
  Lean and Fat
  Lean only
Rump Steak, Grilled:
  Lean and Fat
  Lean only

 = negligible

Grams per 25g/1oz (approx)

	1 2 3 4 5 6 7 8 9 10 11 12 13 14 15 16 17 18 19 20 21 22 23 24 25

Silverside, Salted and
    Boiled:
    Lean and Fat
    Lean only

Sirloin, Roast or Grilled:
    Lean and Fat
    Lean only

Stewing Steak:
    Stewed, Lean and Fat

Topside Roast:
    Lean and Fat
    Lean only

LAMB
Breast, Roast:
    Lean and Fat
    Lean only

Chops, Loin, Grilled:
  Lean and Fat
  Lean and Fat weighed with
    bone
  Lean only
  Lean only weighed with bone
Cutlets, Grilled:
  Lean and Fat
  Lean and Fat weighed with
    bone
  Lean only
  Lean only weighed with bone
Leg Roast:
  Lean and Fat
  Lean only
Scrag and Neck, Stewed:
  Lean and Fat
  Lean only
  Lean only weighed with bone

♦ = negligible

Grams per 25g/1oz (approx)

Scale: 1 2 3 4 5 6 7 8 9 10 11 12 13 14 15 16 17 18 19 20 21 22 23 24 25

Shoulder Roast:
Lean and Fat
Lean only

PORK
Belly Rashers:
Grilled Lean and Fat
Chops, Loin, Grilled:
Lean and Fat
Lean and Fat weighed with bone
Lean only
Lean only weighed with fat and bone
Leg Roast:
Lean and Fat
Lean only

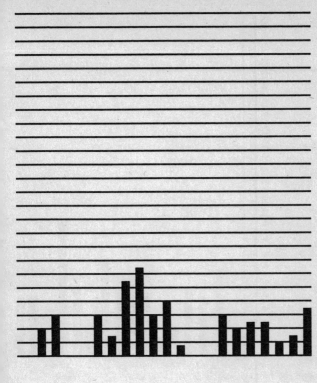

VEAL
Cutlet, Fried
Fillet, Roast

MEATS CANNED
Corned Beef
Ham
Ham and Pork, Chopped
Luncheon Meat
Stewed Steak with Gravy
Tongue
Veal, Jellied

MEAT - COOKED DISHES
Beef Steak Pudding
Beef Stew
Bolognese Sauce
Curried Meat
Hot Pot
Irish Stew
Moussaka

◆ = negligible

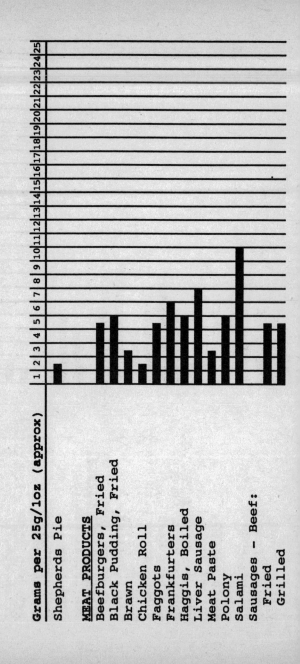

Grams per 25g/1oz (approx)

Shepherds Pie

MEAT PRODUCTS
Beefburgers, Fried
Black Pudding, Fried
Brawn
Chicken Roll
Faggots
Frankfurters
Haggis, Boiled
Liver Sausage
Meat Paste
Polony
Salami
Sausages - Beef:
  Fried
  Grilled

1 2 3 4 5 6 7 8 9 10 11 12 13 14 15 16 17 18 19 20 21 22 23 24 25

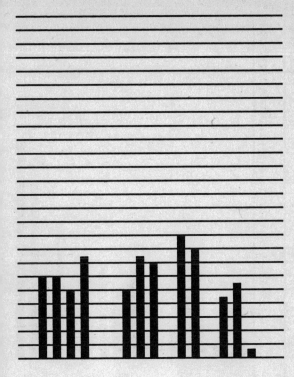

Sausages Pork:
    Fried
    Grilled
    Saveloy
    White Pudding

MEAT AND PASTRY PRODUCTS
Cornish Pasty
Pork Luncheon Meat
Pork Pie
Sausage Roll:
    Flaky Pastry
    Short Pastry
Steak and Kidney Pie:
    Pastry Top only
    Individual
    Turkey Roll

MILK AND MILK SUBSTITUTES

♦ = negligible

Grams per 25g/1oz (approx)

Milk, Cow's:
  Fresh, Whole
  Channel Isles
  Sterilised
  Longlife, UHT Treated
  Fresh, Skimmed
  Shape – semi skimmed
  Condensed, Whole
  Condensed, Skimmed
  Evaporated, Whole
  Dried, Whole
  Dried, Skimmed
Milk, Goats

MINCEMEAT – (fruit)

NUTS
Almonds
Barcelona

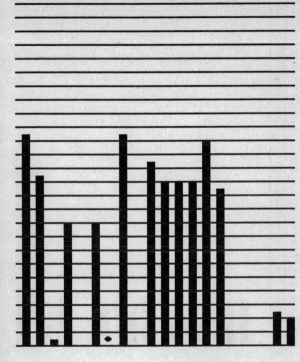

Brazil
Cashews
Chestnuts
Cob or Hazel
Coconut:
   Fresh
   Milk
   Desiccated
Peanuts:
   Dry Roasted
   Fresh
   Roasted and Salted
Peanut Butter
Salted Mixed Nuts
Walnuts

OFFAL
Brain:
   Calf, Boiled
   Lamb, Boiled

◆ = negligible

Grams per 25g/1oz (approx)

Scale: 1 2 3 4 5 6 7 8 9 10 11 12 13 14 15 16 17 18 19 20 21 22 23 24 25

Heart:
- Sheep, Roast
- Ox, Stewed

Kidney:
- Lamb, Fried
- Ox, Stewed
- Pig, Stewed

Liver:
- Calf, Fried
- Chicken, Fried
- Lamb, Fried
- Ox, Stewed
- Pig, Stewed

Oxtail:
- Stewed
- Stewed, weighed with bone

Sweetbread:
- Lamb Fried

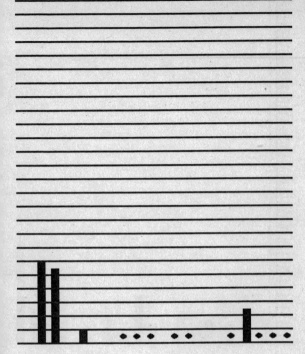

Tongue:
    Lamb, Stewed
    Ox, Boiled
Tripe:
    Stewed

PASTA
Lasagne
Macaroni
Spaghetti, boiled
Spaghetti, canned in Tomato
        Sauce
Tagliatelle

PICKLES
Branston Pickle
Cocktail Olives
Chutney
Piccalilli
Pickle, Sweet

♦ = negligible

Grams per 25g/1oz (approx)

PIZZA

POULTRY

Chicken, Boiled:
  Meat only
  Light Meat
  Dark Meat

Chicken Roast:
  Meat only
  Meat and Skin
  Light Meat
  Dark Meat
  Wing Quarter, weighed with bone
  Leg Quarter, weighed with bone

Duck Roast:
  Meat only
  Meat, Fat and Skin

Scale: 1 2 3 4 5 6 7 8 9 10 11 12 13 14 15 16 17 18 19 20 21 22 23 24 25

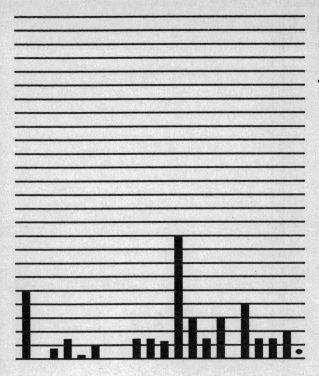

Goose, Roast
Turkey Roast:
  Meat only
  Meat and Skin
  Light Meat
  Dark Meat

PUDDINGS
Angel Delight (made up)
Apple Crumble
Bread and Butter Pudding
Cheesecake
Christmas Pudding
Egg Custard
Dumpling
Fruit Pie with Pastry Top
  and Bottom
Fruit Pie Pastry Top Only
Ice-Cream, Dairy
Ice-Cream, non Dairy
Jelly

♦ = negligible

Grams per 25g/1oz (approx)

Food	1	2	3	4	5	6	7	8	9	10	11	12	13	14	15	16	17	18	19	20	21	22	23	24	25
Lemon Meringue Pie			▇																						
Meringues	•																								
Milk Puddings	▇																								
Rice, Canned	▇																								
Pancakes				▇																					
Queen of Puddings		▇																							
Sponge Pudding				▇																					
Suet Pudding				▇																					
Treacle Tart			▇																						
Trifle	▇																								

PULSES AND LENTILS - Cooked

Food	1	2	3	4	5	6	7	8	9	10	11	12	13	14	15	16	17	18	19	20	21	22	23	24	25
Black Eye Beans	•																								
Butter Beans	•																								
Chick Peas	▇																								
Continental Lentils	•																								
Green Split Peas	•																								
Haricot Beans	•																								
Lentils	•																								

Mung Beans
Red Kidney Beans
Yellow Split Peas

QUICHE LORRAINE

RICE
Cooked
Savoury – Dry Weight

SALAD PRODUCTS
Coleslaw, Low Calorie
Coleslaw, Normal
Shape Coleslaw
Shape 1000 Island Coleslaw
Shape Garlic and Herb
    Coleslaw
Shape Potato Salad
Shape Curried Potato Salad
Shape Chilli Potato Salad

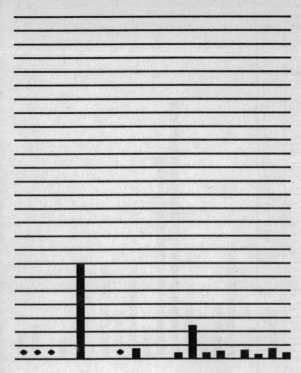

◆ = negligible

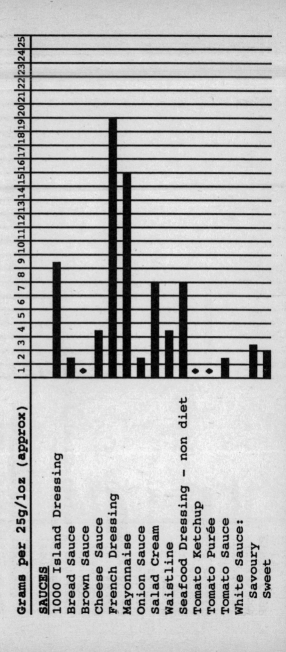

Grams per 25g/1oz (approx)

SAUCES

	1 2 3 4 5 6 7 8 9 10 11 12 13 14 15 16 17 18 19 20 21 22 23 24 25
1000 Island Dressing	
Bread Sauce	
Brown Sauce	
Cheese Sauce	
French Dressing	
Mayonnaise	
Onion Sauce	
Salad Cream	
Waistline	
Seafood Dressing - non diet	
Tomato Ketchup	
Tomato Purée	
Tomato Sauce	
White Sauce:	
Savoury	
Sweet	

SOFT DRINKS
Coca Cola
Grapefruit Juice
Lemonade
Lime Juice Cordial
Lucozade
Orange Drink
Orange Juice
Pineapple Juice
Ribena
Rosehip Syrup
Tomato Juice

SOUPS
Bone and Vegetable Broth
Chicken Cream of:
   Ready to Serve
   Condensed
   Condensed, as Served
Chicken Noodle
Lentil

♦ = negligible

Grams per 25g/1oz (approx)

Scale: 1 2 3 4 5 6 7 8 9 10 11 12 13 14 15 16 17 18 19 20 21 22 23 24 25

Food	Approx. grams per 25g/1oz
Minestrone	•
Mushroom, Cream of	2
Oxtail	1
Tomato, Cream of:	
Ready to Serve	2
Condensed	3
Condensed, as Served	1 •
Vegetable	•

SOYA
Food	Approx. grams per 25g/1oz
Soya, full fat	6
Soya, low fat	3

SUGARS
Food	Approx. grams per 25g/1oz
Glucose Liquid	•
Sugar, all	•
Syrup	•
Treacle	•

VEGETABLES

Ackee, Canned
Artichokes:
  Globe, Boiled
  Jerusalem, Boiled
Asparagus
Aubergine
Avocado
Beans:
  French
  Runner
  Broad
  Butter
  Haricot
  Baked, Canned in Tomato
    Sauce
  Mung, Green Cooked
  Red Kidney
Bean Sprouts
Beetroot
Broccoli Tops

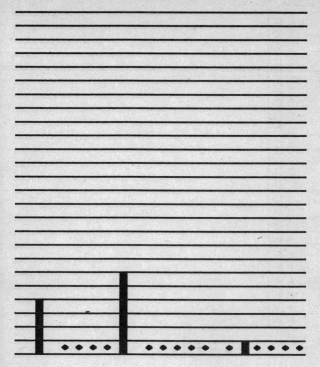

♦ = negligible

Grams per 25g/1oz (approx)

	1	2	3	4	5	6	7	8	9	10	11	12	13	14	15	16	17	18	19	20	21	22	23	24	25
Brussels Sprouts																									
Cabbage:																									
Red																									
Savoy																									
Spring																									
White																									
Winter																									
Carrots																									
Cauliflower																									
Celeriac																									
Celery																									
Chicory																									
Cucumber																									
Horseradish																									
Laverbread																									
Leeks																									
Lentils, Raw																									
Masar Dhal, Cooked																									
Lettuce																									

Marrow
Mushrooms, Raw
Mushrooms, Fried
Mustard and Cress
Okra
Onions all except Fried
Onions, Fried
Parsley
Parsnips
Peas, all kinds
Chick Peas:
    Bengal, Cooked Dhal
    Channa, Dhal
Peppers, Green
Plantain:
    Green, Boiled
    Ripe, Fried
Potatoes:
    Boiled, Baked with/without skins, or Roast, no fat
    Roast, with Fat

♦ = negligible

Grams per 25g/1oz (approx)

	1 2 3 4 5 6 7 8 9 10 11 12 13 14 15 16 17 18 19 20 21 22 23 24 25
Chips, average Home Made	
Chips, Frozen, Fried	
Oven Chips	
Crisps	
Pumpkin	
Radishes	
Salsify	
Seakale	
Spinach	
Spring Greens	
Swedes	
Sweetcorn	
Sweet Potatoes	
Tomatoes	
Tomatoes, Fried	
Turnips	
Watercress	
Yam	

YOGURT (low fat)
Natural
Flavoured
Fruit
Hazelnut
Shape - all flavours
Shape French Style Set Yogurt
Strained Greek Ewe's

YORKSHIRE PUDDING

◆ = negligible

Extra help is available

There are many Rosemary Conley workout videos and audio tapes, all of which are available by mail order. In addition, there is a Hip and Thigh Diet Postal Slimming Course for those who need personal support. For a free list of products and details of the Postal Slimming Course, without obligation, please send a stamped, self-addressed envelope to the address below, marking the envelope MO/PC.

ROSEMARY CONLEY ENTERPRISES
PO BOX 4
MOUNTSORREL,
LOUGHBOROUGH
LEICESTERSHIRE LE12 7LB

Because of the vastly increased volume of work in which I am now involved I regret I am not able always to reply to readers' letters individually. If you have a simple question regarding the diet, I or a member of my personally trained staff will do our best to answer it, but please keep your letter brief and enclose a stamped, self-addressed envelope for a reply. Thank you for your co-operation.